THE
ULTIMATE
BODY
PLAN

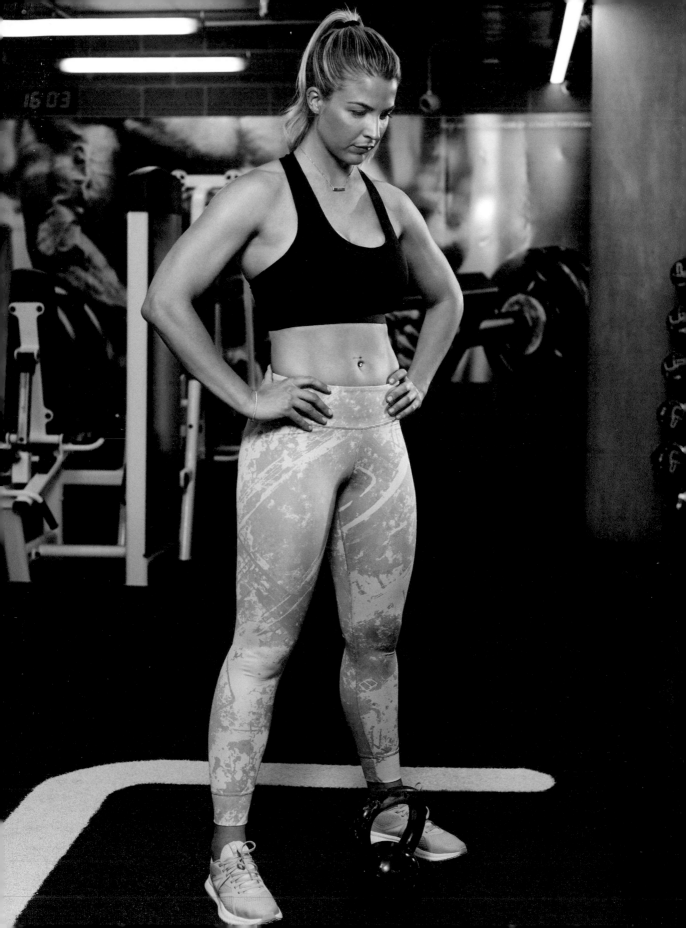

THE ULTIMATE BODY PLAN

75 easy recipes plus workouts
for a leaner, fitter you

GEMMA ATKINSON

Thorsons

Thorsons
An imprint of HarperCollins*Publishers*
1 London Bridge Street
London SE1 9GF

www.harpercollins.co.uk

First published by Thorsons 2018

10 9 8 7 6 5 4 3 2

Text © Gemma Atkinson 2018
Photography © David Cummings: pages 2, 6, 14, 20, 21, 23, 26, 33–42, 54, 138, 158–235; © Martin Poole: pages 53, 57–136, 141–157; photo by Dave J Hogan/Getty Images: page 27; all other images reproduced with permission of the author.

Gemma Atkinson asserts the moral right to be identified as the author of this work

Contributing writer: Jo Usmar
Personal trainer: Steve Chambers, Ultimate Performance Manchester
Exercise programme: Olly Foster www.action-reaction-training.com
Gym: Ultimate Performance Manchester www.upfitness.co.uk
Portrait photography: David Cummings
Stylist: Lucy Denver at Reebok
Hair and make-up: Thembi Mkandla, Bella Campbell and Cinta Miller
Food photography: Martin Poole
Food stylist: Kim Morphew
Prop stylist: Jo Harris
Recipe consultants: Heather Thomas, Olly Foster

A catalogue record of this book is available from the British Library

ISBN 978-0-00-830929-9

Printed and bound at GPS Group

MIX
Paper from
responsible sources
FSC **FSC™ C007454**
www.fsc.org

CONTENTS

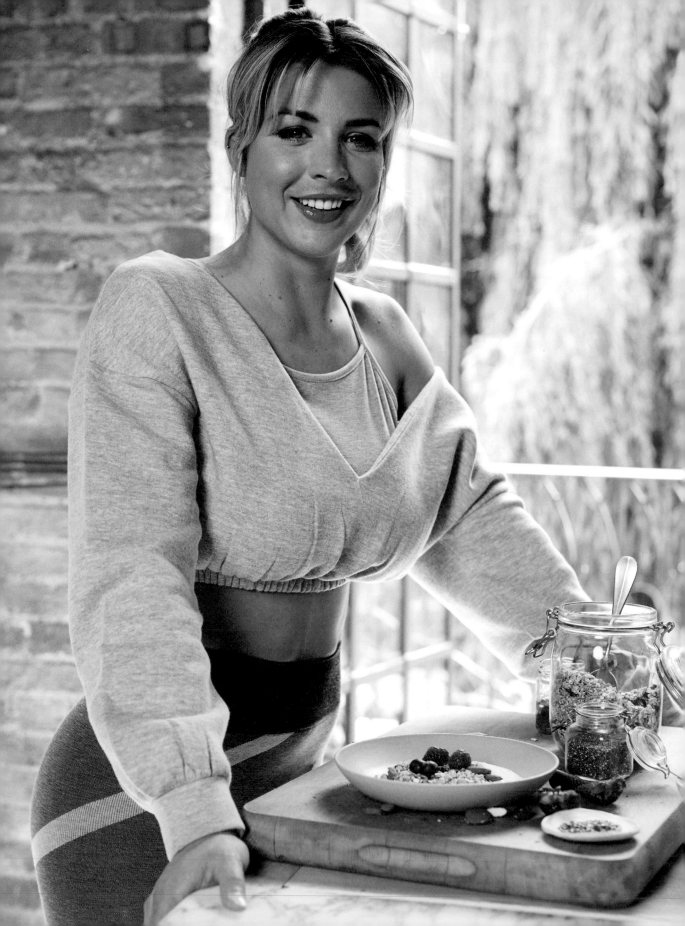

Dear Reader,

Hello and thank you for picking up *The Ultimate Body Plan*. This 12-week nutrition and exercise plan will make you leaner and fitter and give you the body you love. How do I know? Because I did it!

My name is Gemma Atkinson. I'm an actress, radio DJ, model, dog fanatic, pyjama-wearing supermarket-goer and proud Mancunian, who can often be found sweating it out in the gym.

In the last couple of years my life has changed beyond recognition, and, as some of you may have noticed, so has my body. I train. I watch what I eat. I take looking after myself seriously. At 34 years old, I feel more confident about how I look now than I did when I was in my twenties. With that confidence comes so much else: I'm healthier, I've got more energy, my skin is clear and I sleep like a baby (when I want to...).

You may know me as sulky schoolgirl Lisa Hunter from the Channel 4 soap *Hollyoaks*. Or you may recognise me from *Casualty*, *Emmerdale*, *Strictly Come Dancing*, the lads' mags I used to model for, my Hits Radio show, or even solely from the fitness-inspired posts I upload to Instagram. Or perhaps you've never seen me before in your life, but picked up this book because 12 weeks to a shiny new you sounds like something you want to get on board with. However you arrived here – to these pages of my very first book (argh!) – welcome! I'm so excited you're up for making changes, because the plan detailed here transformed my life and it'll do the same for yours too.

I'm really proud that I've found what makes me happy and what makes me feel good, that I've learned how to appreciate my body for what it is and what it can do and that I can share that with others. So many people go their whole lives without feeling good about themselves. You can do this. Just change your environment for 12 weeks and I can guarantee you won't ever want to go back.

By picking up this book you're taking the first step on a journey that will change your life. All you have to do is decide to commit and you'll succeed.

Good luck!

Gemma x

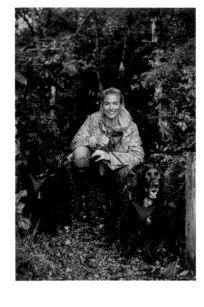

How it all began

So, what inspired me to write this book? Well, since getting my first TV acting role when I was 15 years old (good old grumpy Lisa Hunter), I've spent nearly 20 years having my appearance scrutinised, analysed, criticised, complimented or casually dismissed in the press or online. You know what? I'm fine with it.

At least I am now.

Because since I started training and properly respecting my body and what it can do, I feel AMAZING.

I have learned to not only give zero f***s about any negativity directed my way about how I look, but to actually love my body and truly appreciate the skin I live in (it's true; stop rolling your eyes please). How? By discovering my inner Xena Warrior Princess, inner Jet from *Gladiators* and inner She-Ra (yep, spot the 90s kid). I can chest-press 15kg dumbbells for three sets of ten reps and deadlift 100kg. If you don't understand a word I just wrote, don't worry – I didn't until a few years ago. But I do now, and trust me when I say that challenging my body and understanding how it works has boosted my confidence and self-esteem no end. It's also changed my perspective on everything: ambition, family, friends... even love... Sound a bit dramatic? That's because it is!

This 12-week programme incorporates 75 delicious recipes, carefully curated to give your body what it needs, with monthly phased workouts – both home-based and gym-based, so you can choose what works best for you – that increase in intensity as the weeks go on. There is a ridiculous myth that women shouldn't do weights. Bollocks! Weights are the only way to get truly lean and sculpt your body. This plan will make you fitter, healthier, stronger and leaner (and curvier in places you want curves – hello J Lo bum), but, most importantly, it will totally alter how you see your body. Instead of hating your 'thunder thighs' (a personal one for me – more details on that particular nickname in the next section), you'll credit them for getting you around for 34 years, for being half of your mum and half of your dad, and for being able to do four sets of 20 walking lunges with 15kg dumbbells in each hand.

All I'm asking is that you dedicate 12 weeks – just 12 weeks! that's nothing in the grand scheme of things – to seeing how far you can go and how good you can feel. The results will be dramatic. You'll lose fat, gain muscle, and even see other subtle changes like your skin, hair and nails becoming visibly healthier. Loads of people message me

Since I started training and properly respecting my body and what it can do, I feel AMAZING.

My skin looks good because I eat well, exercise effectively and get proper sleep.

saying, 'What creams do you use on your skin?' Nothing but Egyptian Magic skin cream. My skin looks good because I eat well, exercise effectively and get proper sleep. That's my not-so closely guarded secret!

Follow this plan and you'll see physical changes in just 21 days and discover a whole new attitude to life. If you really throw yourself into this and take it seriously, you'll feel more capable, more positive and more able to deal with whatever comes your way. By the end of the plan, you'll have learned how to break bad habits, how to stop punishing yourself for not being or looking like someone else, and to accept the things you cannot change. We're all different and are built in different ways. This plan is about appreciating your body for what it is, working with it and trying to be the best version of you that you can be, both physically and mentally.

Let's get one thing straight right off: this is not a quick-fix diet plan that promises you'll weigh a certain amount in a few weeks if you starve yourself to near-death and stop doing everything that makes life fun and worth living. I think those plans are unsustainable and bad for you. (Plus, I've always hated that the first three letters of the word diet are 'die' – I think that says it all really.) This plan is a lifestyle change – something that you'll learn to fit into your daily routine that'll overhaul things long-term. The longer you do this, the more your body will adapt and the stronger it will become, so when you do slip up (because hello, that's life), or need a little time off, it's fine, because you'll know exactly how to get back on track. And the best bit is, you'll want to keep at it because you'll feel so much better doing it than not doing it.

Sure, it's easier to carry on watching TV than to work out, but it's also going to be easier putting on that outfit and feeling good about yourself, than putting it on and crying because you feel like absolute crap. In 21 days your stomach and thighs will feel tighter when you sit down, your arms will look more toned, you'll feel less bloated, you'll be sleeping better and you'll have more energy. And that's in just three weeks. Imagine how good you'll feel in 12.

It's time to look after yourself and to stop neglecting your body – it's yours, and if you're lucky, it's going to be with you for a long time. So often people do everything to look after their kids, partner, dogs or mates, while disregarding themselves. It's time to spend some time on you, for you.

Nothing looks better on someone than confidence – and I'm going to help you find that. I'm going to help you feel and look great, so you can rock that bikini with pride, stride into that job interview with your head held high, get over that ex who didn't deserve you, and give a big middle finger to anyone who says it can't be done.

Tomboys and thunder thighs

Growing up, I was a tomboy. My family would wind me up saying if I'd been born first, my parents wouldn't have had another child, because our kid, my elder sister Nina, really was the perfect baby. She slept through the night. She'd say, 'Mummy, dirty hands' and hold them out to be washed. She'd help with the food shopping and the chores. She was just all-round great. Then, seven years later, I arrived. I never slept. When I helped out I would sulk about it, or at least ask for some pocket money in return! I was trying to hustle from the age of 10, ha! I used to go and hide in my dad's pickup truck, lay flat on the trailer and come in covered in mud. Mum would panic whenever I went out as I'd always come home with cuts on my head and scraped knees. Plus, I spent all my time in the garage with my dad and granddad, 'helping' them to build the Caterham Super 7 cars (two-seater sports cars) that my dad raced. I remember him working on this white and silver one for a year and when it was finished he'd take me and my friends, one-by-one, for a ride in it on Sundays. Whenever he raced, we'd make a weekend of it, piling into the caravan to go watch him with our packed lunches. Of course, this meant a lot of the time I was covered in oil and grease and I absolutely loved it!

I was into *Ghostbusters* and *Teenage Mutant Ninja Turtles*. Barbies and stuff? No chance. I had a WWE wrestling belt and ring instead. I had all the wrestling stickers and books. People still say to me actually, 'You should be a WWE Diva', and if anyone from the wrestling world is reading this – sign me up!

Because I was into kick-ass women – the Xenas, the Jets and the She-Ras – whenever there was a chance to do sports at school, I took it. I did hockey, netball, rounders, athletics and trampolining. I also ran the 100m and was the fourth leg of the relay for local club Manchester Girls. I absolutely loved it for the comradery, being part of a team, and getting stronger, even though I didn't come first (although at the time I clearly thought I was Sally Gunnell).

That's where the nickname 'Thunder Thighs' came from: the fact that I was both a runner and had big legs. At the time it never bothered me because it was only ever said in a funny, affectionate way, and it never stopped me from doing what I loved. But I think subconsciously it may have got under my skin a little because I do remember thinking, 'My legs are quite muscly, I don't really want to get them out,' and I'd always wear trousers at school when we were allowed to, during the winter. Plus, wearing trousers also meant I

INTRODUCTION

I was into *Ghostbusters* and *Teenage Mutant Ninja Turtles*. Barbies and stuff? No chance.

> All the things I've done and achieved in my life resulted from that very first audition which I got because my mum believed in me.

didn't have to bother shaving my legs! (Shaving – what a total, utter and absolute ballache.)

That brief history might give you some idea as to why I responded the way I did when my mum picked me up from school one day when I was 15 and, instead of taking me to the dentist like she'd said, took me to a modelling agency. 'No way! ABSOLUTELY NOT!' I roared as we pulled up. Which is exactly what she'd known I'd do, which is why she'd kept it secret. Me? Modelling? I'd got hairy legs and didn't own a single lipstick. I lived in trackies and dungarees. 'Listen, a few people have seen family photos of you and said I should enrol you here. You never know what it'll lead to,' she said, ushering me in, while I mentally prepared my escape route.

So we turned up at Manchester Modelling Agency (MMA) and I genuinely couldn't believe I was there rather than at home on my Playstation. Surprisingly, bearing in mind the confused, gormless look on my face, the agency signed me up. They took some photos, made me a portfolio and sent us on our way. I didn't think anything more about it. Then, about a month later, they called saying there was a casting for *Hollyoaks*. The soap was looking for a grumpy schoolgirl called Lisa Hunter and the agency thought I'd be a great fit! Charming. But I did the audition and two hours later they told me I'd got the job.

And that's where it all started, and I've got my mum to thank for everything! She was spot on. I loved it as soon as I did it. But had she told me her idea before arriving at MMA, I wouldn't have gone. All the things I've done and achieved in my life resulted from that very first audition which I got because my mum believed in me. Thanks, Mum!

Calendar girls

I'd never acted properly before. Drama classes at school mostly consisted of sitting in the common room chatting for an hour a week. I'd also never even seen *Hollyoaks*! When I got the job, my family and friends were way more excited than I was, saying, 'Oh! You're going to get to work with Gary Lucy and James Redmond!' while I had no idea who they were. I didn't realise it was a big deal. It was only after the show came out and people started stopping me on the street asking if I was on the TV that I thought, 'Ah okay, people other than my mates watch this'.

I did an acting course before shooting my first scene and found the whole thing exciting, but I think being so young made me quite blasé about it. Mum wouldn't let me extend the initial contract until

Clockwise from top left: Chilling with my dad. I always felt safe up there on his shoulders; Rocking my one-piece in Tenerife. I'm fuming because Mum made me cut my hair short the week before; Helping Dad build our back fence! I was probably getting right in his way, right under his feet and right on his nerves, but still he always let me help; Fifth year of high school in my PE kit. My fringe hair-sprayed within an inch of its life!; My first BMX. I fell off at least 20 times in the first week learning to do wheelies... But I always got back on!

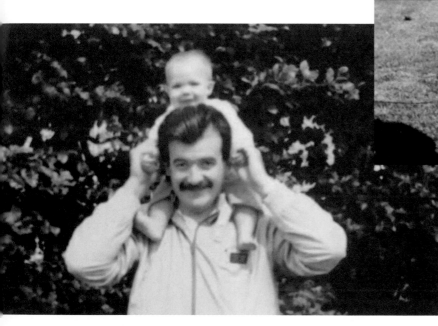

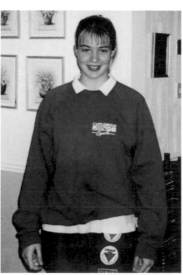

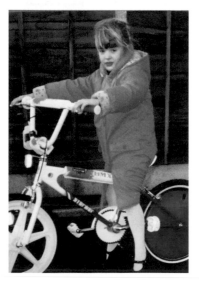

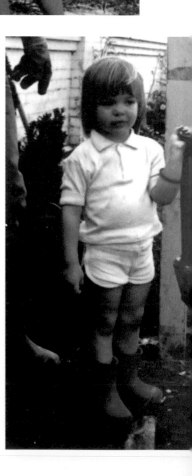

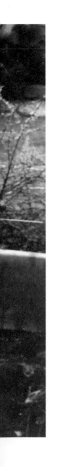

I'd passed my GCSEs though, so I got the grades I needed to study sports therapy, which is what I'd always wanted to do, then I signed up to *Hollyoaks* full-time for a year. That ended up turning into seven altogether; five on the main show and two on the spin-offs *Hollyoaks: Let Loose* and *Hollyoaks: In the City*.

I always joke with my friends now that it's a good job social media wasn't around when we were at school. I didn't have that extraordinary pressure young people face now to look a certain way. I remember the first moment I ever felt truly insecure about how I looked: when we shot a *Hollyoaks* calendar in Ibiza when I was 17, I was with beautiful women who were two or three years older than me, were quite slim and also more physically developed, like the lovely Sarah Dunn who played Mandy, and Elize du Toit who played Izzy. When I saw the photos I thought, 'Oh gosh, I don't look like these other girls. I look heavier, my roots are quite bad, and my nails are all bitten'. They'd all had manicures and pedicures and their hair done, but, because I was young, I thought that's just how they looked all the time. It didn't occur to me that they had got their hair and nails done specially. It was the first time I really questioned my appearance.

Earlier that year, in April 2002, my dad passed away. It was, and still is, the single biggest thing that's ever happened to me in my life and it hit me massively hard. While I didn't go off the rails as such, I did stop looking after myself a bit. I'd think nothing of going out and sinking five shots of vodka of an evening. My friends and I would go out on Friday and Saturday nights drinking, have a McDonald's on the Saturday and a Chinese takeaway on the Sunday. None of us would ever think, 'I'm going to feel like crap tomorrow,' or 'We're going to get fat'. We just did it. It's only when I look back now that I realise, 'that's why my face was puffy, my skin used to break out, and why I didn't sleep very well. I mean, we used to get a flight to Magaluf on a Friday, come back on Sunday and then head straight to work on the Monday. We weren't on our phones trying to get our best angles to upload to Instagram, we just let ourselves be and we needed that. I needed that. That whole period was full of laughter and love.

But it all took its toll, meaning I definitely didn't look my best when shooting that *Hollyoaks* calendar. It was, I think, my very first insight into what social media is now – being forced to compare myself to other women. I spent that whole week in Ibiza thinking, 'This is so embarrassing. I look chubby, young and stupid.' I even wondered if the press people would regret me being in it. Then, when it came to promotion, the agency said to me, '*The Daily Star*, *The Sun* and *The Mirror* all want to use your shot to advertise the calendar.' My photo – out of all of them. I couldn't believe it. Many of the papers did use my photo. Then, off the back of that, the agency said, 'The response has been great. We want you to do your own calendar.' So I shot my

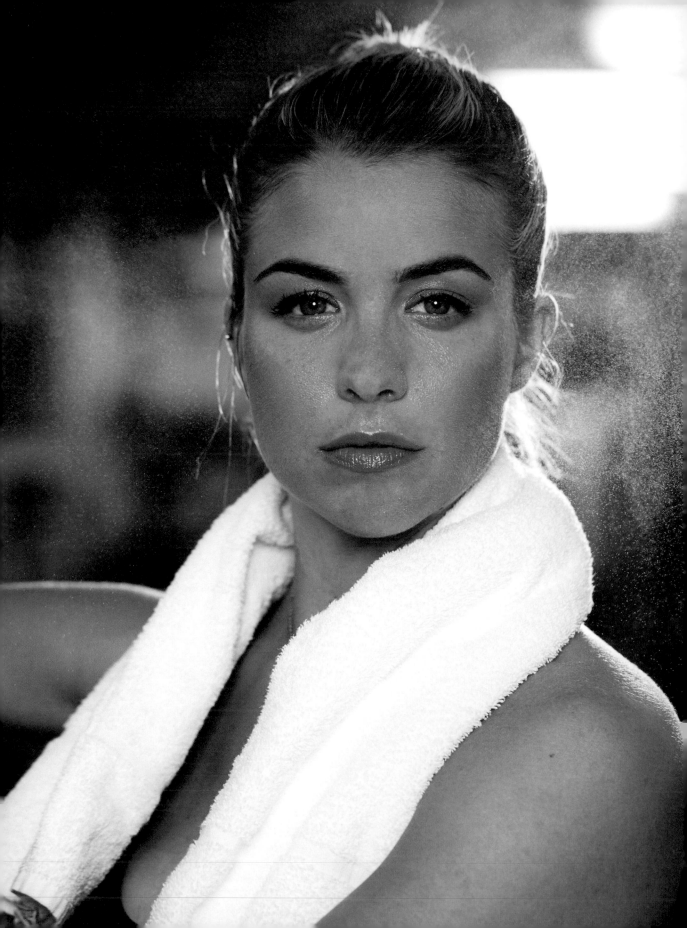

own, the whole time thinking, 'Is anyone actually going to buy this?' But then the lads' mags picked up on it and it basically kick-started my modelling career. Which just goes to show, you know? I spent an entire week – and all the lead-up to the calendar being released – panicking about it. Panicking that I didn't look right, that I was too big and un-groomed, too much of a tomboy; that I didn't look like everyone else. Yet off the back of that I ended up shooting five or six of my own calendars. Something great came from a week of stressing over something that was all in my own head. It taught me that we never know the full story, that we can look at an Instagram post and think, 'Oh, look at her with her perfect life', not realising she's spent the day doubled over with anxiety about something or other.

That was a big lesson for me – how comparing yourself to others can send you down a spiral of self-doubt. And, as my modelling career took off and papers and magazines started becoming interested in my personal life, I'd have a few more lessons coming my way…

The heartbreak diet

I started going to the gym when I was 20, but had absolutely no idea what I was doing. I'd run on the treadmill for half an hour every day and do some dumbbell curls and that was it. I'd also read somewhere that cutting out carbs was the thing to do, so I did that… and was always totally knackered. My skin turned grey, my hair stopped growing properly and I looked awful. I didn't have a clue about training or nutrition, wasn't getting the energy or nutrients I needed, and was just flogging my body on this treadmill. I lost a lot of weight quickly due to crash dieting and endless cardio and, as is often the case when that happens, my boobs were the first things to go.

I'd always had big boobs – they run in the family – but I was soon saying to my mum, 'Look at my boobs, they look so saggy, they're awful,' as I could actually pick up the skin where they'd deflated, like balloons. During photoshoots I would have to wear push-up bras because I didn't feel comfortable in a bikini any more. I became really self-conscious. I just didn't look like *me* any more.

I told my mum I wanted a boob job. 'Don't be ridiculous!' she cried. 'If you think they're saggy now, wait until you have two kids like I have!' She joked about it, but soon realised how serious I was and how down I felt. We'd go shopping and I'd stand miserably in the changing room because clothes didn't hang right or like I wanted

> I started going to the gym when I was 20, but had absolutely no idea what I was doing.

> It was part of my career to do photoshoots in a bikini – that was a big part of how I made my living. I couldn't cover up and I didn't want to feel crappy about it.

them to. She eventually agreed to come with me to meet a doctor at Transform, the plastic surgery clinic. He explained the process and showed me photos – I think Mum was secretly hoping that would put me off, but it didn't at all. I was determined... and so I did it. Just before my 22nd birthday I got my old boobs back(!) and moved to Mum's while I recovered from the surgery.

It was part of my career to do photoshoots in a bikini – that was a big part of how I made my living. I couldn't cover up and I didn't want to feel crappy about it. So I didn't – and still don't – regret having them done for a moment. I immediately felt like the old me again. I didn't do it for anyone else, I did it for me. To make me feel good, because my body had changed shape and I wanted to feel confident again.

When I was 22, I met Premier League footballer Marcus Bent and we started dating. It was my first 'high-profile' relationship. I was naïve about what that meant at the time and so was totally unprepared for the press interest. During the time I was working with the lads' mags, I tried to remain as unaffected by the press coverage and constant analysis of my life and looks as possible. When I hadn't been living in the heart of the tabloid loop, it was easy-ish... but that all changed when I met Marcus. There were articles guessing how long it would last, wondering whether we were going to move in together, get engaged or have a baby. We'd be snapped when we were out and people would comment on what I was wearing or whether there was something wrong if we weren't together.

We got engaged in 2008, a few months after I got back from filming *I'm a Celebrity Get Me Out of Here*, but split later that year, just before my 24th birthday in November. I found it incredibly tough, even though it was my decision. Marcus was extremely kind and caring, but something just wasn't sitting right. Yes, I could have stayed in an okay relationship and had no financial worries due to his profession, but I'd grafted my whole life to get where I was (moving out to live on my own at 17), so I had my own money and besides, that's never been a driving factor for me in a relationship. I wanted the little things money can't buy – glances across a crowded room and loving Post-it notes left on a mirror. I remember Mum saying, 'Gem, do you see yourself with this person forever?' and I said, 'I don't know', and she said, 'Well, you categorically cannot marry him then because with the right man, you wouldn't think twice about answering yes to that question.' That was it, I knew I had to end it.

I was devastated. It can be as hard to break up with someone as it is to be broken up with, especially when that person has done nothing wrong. You've got this overwhelming sense of guilt and then the worry over whether you've done the right thing. I'd wake up in the morning

> It dawned on me that I'd rather feel good than look a certain way.

and for a split second feel fine... then I'd remember what'd happened and feel physically sick. I was walking hunched over because if I stood upright my stomach would hurt. I couldn't eat much and so lost even more weight. Then the weirdest thing happened. People started telling me how great I looked! My eyes were hollow, I was shaky and anxious, my skin was grey and my hair was lank, yet just because I was skinny, people said, 'Oh God, you look fab! What's your secret?' I wanted to reply, 'Heartbreak and misery, pal', but of course I didn't. I said, 'Thank you', while thinking, 'Do you really think I look good? Because I feel like absolute crap. What does that say about what you think looks good?'

I was dealing with all of that, plus the split was being played out all over the media. It was surreal. Especially when every article focused on what *I* must have done wrong – that there must have been something wrong with me. It all added to my stress, anxiety and self-doubt.

I was filming the live-action segment for the game *Command & Conquer* around this time and you could see my ribs in pictures. There's a promotional image of me in the uniform and my hands dwarf my waist, my legs look like drainpipes and my cheekbones are nearly cutting my skin. The thing is, it is a glamorous photo – I'm all made up and posing like a professional. You could look at it and think, 'She looks nice,' but because I know how I felt when it was taken, I see it now and think, 'I *never* want to look like that again'.

At the time I said to Mum, 'God, if I feel like this every day, life's going to be horrific'. She said, 'Oh Gemma, I've got news for you. This won't be the last time you go through heartbreak, but it also won't be the last time you get over it. You *will* get through it. And then you'll get heartbroken again and get through it again.' It's totally true, but when you're in that state yourself, you can't see it or hear it. You think it's the end of the world – that you're going to end up an old spinster living alone with ten dogs.

While everyone was being so complimentary about how great I looked all I could think was, 'Hang on, if I look great now, didn't I look good before?' and the insecurity cycle cranked up again. That's when it struck me, how twisted it all was – that the only reason I looked supposedly 'great' was because I wasn't eating or sleeping and felt horrendous. How is that something to aspire to?

It dawned on me that I'd rather *feel* good than look a certain way. I could try to get over the break-up, sort myself out, and yes, be a bit heavier, but be happier and healthier. I thought, 'Sack what I look like – I just need to feel happy again', because yes, people can look a certain way, but you have no idea what they're going through below the surface. It's like, 'Your insides are rotting, but you look great! Heartbreak's the secret! Just get shat on and you'll look lovely!'

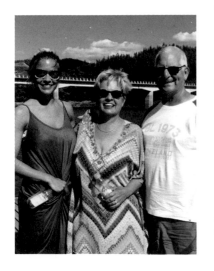

With my mum Sandra and stepdad Peter. Holidays with them are still so much fun.

Heartbreak is something most people have gone through or will go through. My mum and dad divorced when I was ten and my mum has told me since that it was the hardest thing she's ever had to do. She said, 'I would have left sooner but you were so young. I couldn't do that to you.' But I said, 'What about yourself, Mum? Why would you stay with Dad if you weren't compatible any more?' She said, 'When you have kids yourself you'll understand.' And some of my friends have stayed with men that weren't right for them and I've thought, 'But you're miserable and wanting to kiss other lads at the weekend when you're drunk because you're so unhappy. How can that be better than leaving? Isn't it better for kids not to live with two sad parents?'

Bottom line is: we have no idea what anyone's going through or dealing with. People could look at pictures of me at the time and think I was on top of the world. Work was going well, I looked 'great', I was young, single and free. Supposedly. When actually I was incredibly unhappy.

When things weren't getting any better, my sister Nina sat me down and said, 'You lost Dad five years ago and you dealt with that – and that's the hardest thing any young girl can deal with. So who the hell is an ex-boyfriend in comparison to Dad?' I thought, 'Oh my god, she's right! If I can get through losing Dad – a man who loved me unconditionally and who I assumed would always be around – I can get through losing a guy I've spent two or three years with.' It made me realise that I was stronger than I knew. That although I might think, 'I can't cope with this', I can. I've got through 34 years of both my best and my worst days and I'm still standing.

I had to channel those thoughts again when things kicked off in the press in exactly the same way after I called off my engagement to Liam Richards in 2013. Actually, that time was worse because they now had *two* 'failed engagements' to pin on me. Liam and I were together for three and a bit years, but split because we were both working so hard we rarely saw each other during the last year. The headlines screamed: 'She has the career, she has this and that, but she can't find love!' Or 'What's wrong with Gemma? Why can't she hold on to a man?' All the time I was thinking, 'But *I* ended it! Maybe I didn't want to settle for something that wasn't right?' Mum said, 'You're getting stressed about something you have no control over. Will them saying this about you matter in five years? No. So why waste five minutes on it then?' That five years-five minutes rule is one I've carried with me throughout my life.

Bottom line is: we have no idea what anyone's going through or dealing with.

> I shouldn't want to get fit to look a certain way, but to feel a certain way. Looking good means nothing if you don't feel good.

Working things out

I still assumed that to be fit the aim was to see numbers drop off the scales. That if I exercised like a demon, I'd look as slim as I did when I was heartbroken, but actually feel great too, rather than wanting to crawl into a hole and cry. But lo-and-behold that didn't happen. No matter how many miles I sweated away on the treadmill or half-hearted dumbbell curls I did, I was still a 5ft 9in woman with muscly legs and broad shoulders. Who'd have thought it, huh? The saddest thing was that I hated my body for it. I was still convinced that to look good, and to look fit, I needed to be smaller – somehow less than I was now. It never occurred to me not to want to get smaller.

Everything changed for me when I started exercising with personal trainer Olly Foster in 2014 at the Ultimate Performance gym in Mayfair when I was working in London. Olly said to me, 'If you could look like anyone, who would it be?' and I said right away, 'Kylie Minogue. She's tiny and petite. She looks great.' He looked me straight in the eye and said, 'You are NEVER going to look like Kylie Minogue. NEVER. You probably looked like Kylie Minogue when you were 12 years old. Let's be realistic.' My jaw dropped. How could he say that?! I was incredibly offended. It was this man's job to *make* me look like Kylie Minogue.

But then I looked around that gym – at all the women weight-lifting and loving it – and realised they weren't using their bodies to look a specific way, they were using them to improve their health, posture, stamina and mental outlook. To improve everything. They were putting looks aside and prioritising how they felt. All different shapes and sizes, all mucking in, grunting and sweating and looking like total badasses! Then it hit me: of course I'm never going to look like Kylie Minogue. It's ridiculous! And nor should I want to, because I'm simply not built that way.

'Oh my God…,' I said, and sat down, kind of stunned, as Olly started working out a programme for me. It's like someone telling you, 'The entire way you see yourself is messed up' and realising they're right. Olly said, 'You've got really strong legs, maybe we could up the weight and you could use them more', and again I was speechless. Instead of saying, 'Let's try to slim down your thighs', he wanted me to make them more muscly?! Hell yes he did. He understood that my 'thunder thighs' could be a good thing. A great thing even. That my body could work in my favour. That instead of trying to be incredibly thin, having drainpipe legs and a pancake bum, I could have strong legs that would carry me further and faster, below a curvy bum.

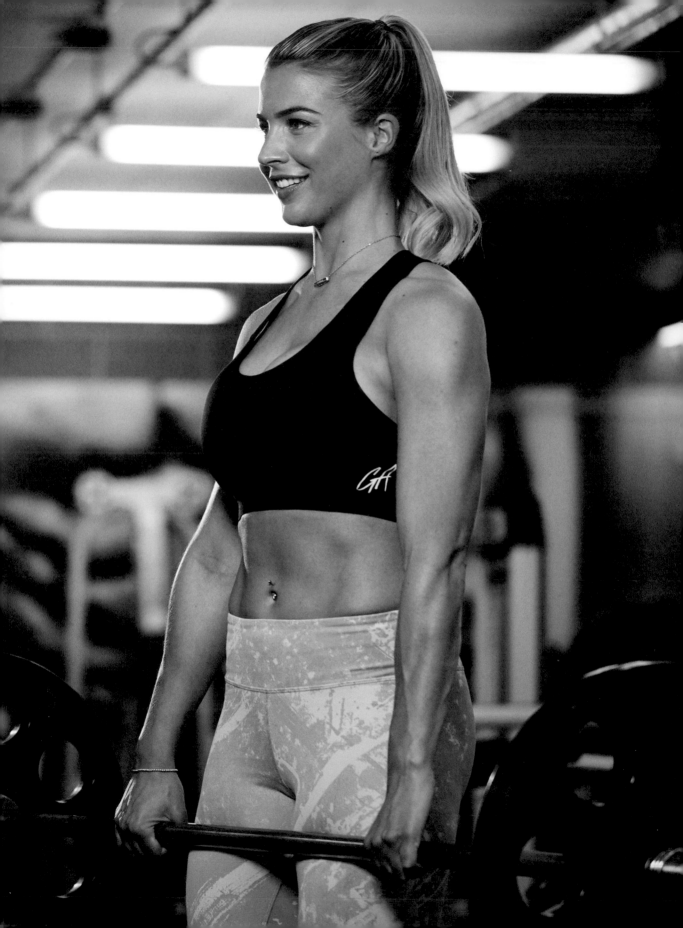

I realised that before now, I'd not only not been using my body to its best advantage, I'd been actively working against it, punishing it for looking the way it did, trying to bully it into being smaller, weighing less, being less. While all the time, all these women in the gym were doing the total opposite.

Think about that for a moment: think about how much you punish your body – treating it badly, hating on it – for not looking like something or someone else. You will look your absolute best – not my best or Kylie's best – when you accept what you cannot change and start working with your body, not against it. I learned an incredibly important lesson that day – I shouldn't want to get fit to *look* a certain way, but to *feel* a certain way. Looking good means nothing if you don't feel good.

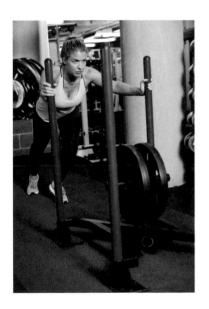

Good things come to women who weight(lift)

Repeat after me: 'weight training will not make me look like a man!' You won't become 'too big' by lifting weights. Women have nowhere near the amount of testosterone they'd need to 'bulk up' to the point that they look masculine. All weight training will do is make you leaner and fitter so you'll still look and feel like a woman, but a warrior woman who can carry all her own bags, thanks very much.

Here are just a few of the benefits of resistance training for women:
1) **It burns more fat.** Yes, it's true that while you're actually performing the exercise you're burning fewer calories weight-lifting than you would doing two hours on the cross-trainer (no, thank you). However, you're actually increasing your metabolic rate, which means you'll be burning more calories for longer afterwards.
2) **You can eat more.** Your muscles will get denser and bigger, so you'll need to eat more to maintain them. Or, looking at it the other way, you can handle a lot more calories. Result.
3) **You'll get stronger bones.** The pressure weight training puts on your bones encourages your body to invest in making them stronger and sturdier. This counteracts the natural propensity for women's bone density to decrease from their 30s onwards.
4) **Your immune system will thank you.** People who lift tend to have better eating habits and better quality of sleep, lower stress levels

and improved circulation, all of which makes you healthier, period.

5) **You'll feel like a combination of Xena, Jet and She-Ra.**

Please remember that the photos you see of me working out in the gym are taken when my muscles are swollen with blood to help me lift the weights. That's why people look pumped during workouts: their muscles are literally 'pumped up'. Bodybuilders and fitness models go out of their way to look bigger and more defined on shoots or at shows, enhancing their muscles (and even making their veins 'pop') through a careful diet, dehydration and fake tan. People can see those images and think, 'I'll look like that all the time if I do weights, even just at the shops!' You absolutely won't. You'll just look toned. Lifting weights won't make you 'butch' or 'manly'; it'll make you more confident, energetic, stronger, leaner, fitter and happier.

Struggling, sweating and swearing

I started training with Olly properly in 2014 and, because I was now training with direction, the changes I went through – both physical and mental – were pretty much immediate. It's not just the natural high that comes from exercising, but eating right also has a huge impact on your mood and body and therefore behaviour. Once you start something good, your body craves it and you feel better for having taken action. I had not only found one of the best personal trainers around, but a great boyfriend too! Olly and I were together for around two years and I'm happy to say we're still mates to this day.

I started posting videos and pictures of my workouts on Instagram and saw how I was able to connect with people in a positive way. Lots of people were into the fact that I was working out to feel good first, and look good second. For that reason I've made it my mission to always be open and honest, both about how I feel and how I look.

Then the trolls arrived. The keyboard warriors who spend all day sitting alone in their parents' basement venting about others because they've got nothing else going on. Lads message me and say, 'You've gone too far, you look like a man' and I'll reply and say, 'Well, lift heavier and maybe you will too!' Yes, that kind of stuff makes me angry, but I'll take a moment and choose to react differently – I actually try to take those comments as compliments now. I mean, at the end of the day, they're still looking, aren't they? If they weren't interested, jealous or annoyed they wouldn't be doing it. No one else's opinion should have the power to make you happy or not. You

Ignore the naysayers and people who don't want to support you, and cut yourself some goddamn slack.

can't control other people's actions, but you can control how you react to them. You can either wallow or brush it off.

My plan from the start has always been to just be me. We all look different, we all have crap days and we all slip up: welcome to the club – there's seven billion of us in it. I want to show that if I can do this, you can too. Commit to looking after yourself, get to know your own body, take social media with a pinch of salt, be honest about your intentions, ignore the naysayers and people who don't want to support you, and cut yourself some goddamn slack.

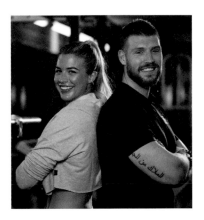

Evil Steve

The Ultimate Body Plan

While my training now had more focus and my aims had changed (no more Kylie hang-ups!), when the summer of 2017 rolled around, I knew I wanted to give myself a new challenge. Olly and I had split up totally amicably in 2016 and I was training back home at the Manchester branch of Ultimate Performance. I was still hosting my radio show, but had just left *Emmerdale* where I'd played Carly Hope for around two years. I absolutely loved the job and the people there, but wanted to change things up. But while I was still hitting the gym, I'd got into a bit of a training rut. So I signed up to the gym's 12-week training plan that promised to transform both your body and your mindset, and started working with personal trainer, Steve Chambers. He soon became known as Evil Steve!

I didn't have a holiday booked or want to get in shape for a specific event, I just wanted to challenge myself. I was seriously curious to see what my body and mind were capable of. Plus, I respond well to stricter routines. It's when you're left to your own devices that you half-heartedly do some weights before heading home and eating three bags of crisps.

This plan is 100% focused on feeling great rather than on vanity. You're far more likely to stick with something if you're doing it for sustainable long-term results (to feel great) than to hit a certain number on the scales (like some faddy diets promise) because, if you don't reach that goal you'll feel like crap. More often than not, even if you do reach it you still feel rubbish because you're not dealing with the cause of your feelings, both mental and physical – bad diet, poor sleep, stress, low self-esteem, lack of energy etc. You're just dealing with what you think is a symptom (weight). You'll then keep punishing your body because you won't know how to feel better, constantly moving the goalposts: 'I'm now a size 8, but I still feel exhausted, run-down, stressed and unhappy. Maybe I'll feel better at a size 6.' No, you won't. This plan offers a total lifestyle overhaul with no unrealistic expectations to falter under. In

In feeling stronger and more positive, you'll be in the best position to take on everything – with looking great a happy side effect.

feeling stronger and more positive, you'll be in the best position to take on everything – with looking great a happy side effect.

The plan meant I had to start cooking and prepping meals in advance, which you will too. People can feel daunted by this, but you can make time for it. If you're serious about change, you'll get up 15 minutes earlier to make your breakfast, or put aside a couple of hours on a Sunday to prep your food for the next few days like I do. Once you get into the routine of it, it becomes second nature. Also, I find it extremely motivating to remember that I'm eating to fuel my muscles, to feel great for the rest of the day. Cutting out rubbish that makes you feel sluggish isn't a chore when you can really feel the results.

So, on day one of the plan, I put my leggings and crop top on and looked in the mirror. I took the top photo opposite (taking progress photos is part of the programme; see page 167) and thought, 'Right, this is how you look now. You've had 32 years on these feet, these legs, looking how you do, feeling how you do. Now it's just 12 weeks to see where it can go and what you can do!' I really psyched myself up for it, getting into the mindset of an athlete before a fight.

The transformation

The first week of the 12-week programme was horrendous. Horrific. The worst. I felt sick, I was shaking and dripping with sweat. 'God, I can't do this,' I thought. 'I want to quit. I want to die.'

But I didn't quit. I didn't die.

What I did do was lose fat, which proved I'd had it to lose in the first place. My body was responding immediately to working out, and after 3 weeks I'd lost 1.5% of my body fat. But it was actually more the mental changes that struck me first. I started feeling proud of myself – knowing I'd sweated, had had a good session and burned loads of calories. Something changed in my body language – my shoulders went down and my chin up and I even walked with more confidence. Plus, I started sleeping better. I already found myself waking up, checking my phone and seeing it was ten minutes before my alarm was due to go off. I wasn't waking feeling sluggish, exhausted or bloated as I'd had a good meal the night before.

Three weeks in, I noticed more definition in my arms. When I sat down my stomach and thighs stayed tight. My entire body was getting leaner and I felt much more energetic. Friends and family also started seeing changes, which is always a huge motivator.

Depending on your fitness levels to start with, your results at

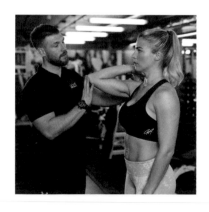

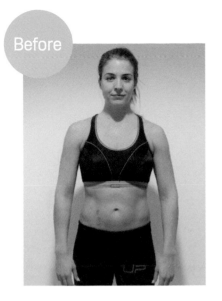

Before I started the Ultimate Body Plan

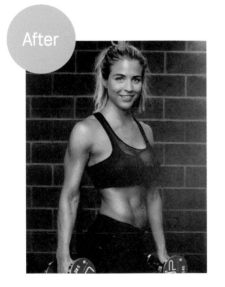

After 12 weeks I'd lost 13lbs and 5% of my body fat.

this stage will probably be even more dramatic than mine were. If you stick to the plan 100% it'll be a shock to the system and you'll shed weight and body fat. However, be warned – you may still be craving the sweet stuff. They say it takes between two to three weeks to cleanse your palette. Keep going! Push through. Your body is essentially detoxing so your skin may actually break out as it gets rid of all the toxins – but then, once they're out and if you keep at it, at around this point your skin will really start to glow!

These changes will spur you on. Your body wants to get better, it wants to get healthier, so as soon as you start nourishing it and treating it well, it'll respond, like it's saying 'thank you'.

Week five was a strange one for me because I actually put some weight back on, hitting around 11 stone – fine for someone of my height with broad shoulders. So don't panic if you put on weight! People can read that I weigh 11 stone and freak out, but I was losing a lot of body fat while gaining muscle mass. So many factors affect women's weight – everything from eating more salt, where you are in your menstrual cycle, and even the weather! (As we tend to drink more water when it's hot.) I felt great, was leaner, my clothes fit better and I was as healthy as I'd ever been. Instead of losing weight, I was aiming to beat my personal bests every week. If I could lift one more rep on a Tuesday than I did on a Monday, I knew I was progressing. I felt amazing, while looking completely different to what was considered 'perfect' in the public eye, or what was considered beautiful by most people. Yes, some magazines think I should be a size 8, but I'm simply not built that way. I'm a size 10–12, but I can squat 90kg.

About midway through the 12-week programme I was asked to be a contestant on *Strictly Come Dancing*, the biggest show on national telly. I told Becca, my agent, that I didn't think it was the right time and I'd like her to turn it down. I was happy with my life the way it was. I loved working on the radio show, I was training hard and I had time for friends and family. For the first time in a long time, there was no press intrusion in my life. I wasn't in the public eye as much and I was really enjoying that.

During week seven I went on holiday with some mates and didn't put a sarong on to walk from the pool to the bar as I felt 100% comfortable in my bikini now. I also had no desire to binge just because I was on holiday – I didn't want to throw away all my hard work. So I took a skipping rope with me, downloaded some HIIT workouts onto my phone before I left, did lots of swimming and went on big walks along the beach. I ate healthy meals and had some treats, but was surprised by how much I didn't want to eat crap, drink loads and sit on my butt all day – not because I felt I had to keep to the plan, but because doing all this had made me feel so good.

It's a strange process actually – realising that you feel incredible.

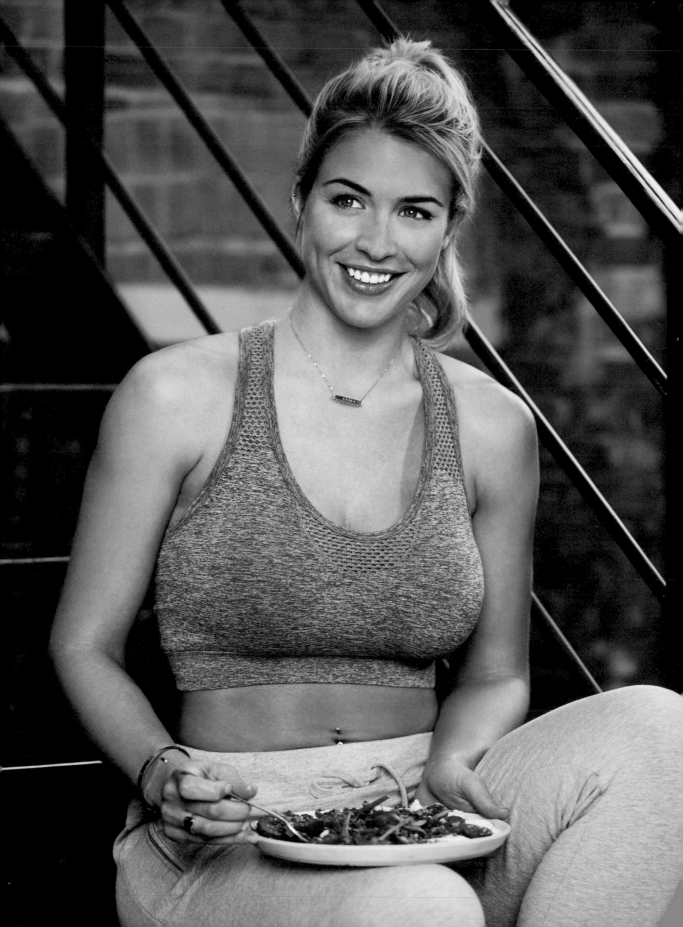

Noticing that you're waking up feeling energetic and determined rather than uncomfortable and tired. I find working out very therapeutic; whether you're doing HIIT or weights, your head goes somewhere else. Some of my best ideas come to me when I'm exercising. You have space and time to yourself – often the only time of day you get that.

At the end of the 12 weeks I took my final set of progress photos and actually got quite teary. The results were shocking – in a good way. I still looked very feminine, but a lot leaner, a lot less body fat. My skin was way clearer. My hair had grown faster and thicker and so had my nails. Even my eyes looked brighter. While my weight had fluctuated on the plan, overall I had lost 13lbs and 5% of my body fat. I felt amazing and was so proud of myself. I'd put my body through so much with fad diets and gruelling gym punishments, and I'd put myself through so much mentally trying to get over men and dealing with guilt and regrets, that I'd really neglected my body. I felt this intense gratitude that I was able to nourish it and look after it and heal it, so to speak.

Strictly come laughing

I think I must be the only contestant in the history of *Strictly Come Dancing* to put *on* weight during the show. But how did I end up waltzing on the sparkliest dancefloor on TV after turning it down? It was all down to Oprah. No, really.

After I'd finished the 12-week plan, I went on Jason Vale's Juice Retreat in Portugal. I go every year to detox, unwind and re-set. Each guest is given a book in their room when they check in and that year I was given Oprah Winfrey's biography. I picked it up and the first page that opened had a single quote on it, from a song by Lee Ann Womack. Of all things, it was about choosing to dance if you have the chance.

Now, I'm a big believer in signs, chance and circumstance and all that, but even if I wasn't, there was no denying that was a bit weird. I showed my mum, who'd come with me, and she simply said, 'Get Becca on the phone', so I rang and said, 'Let's do it.' I knew *Strictly* was a huge opportunity and I also knew I was in a far better headspace to deal with being back on primetime telly again. I was more confident, self-assured and mature. I felt like I could handle it. Thank you, 12-week programme!

But that didn't mean I wasn't nervous as hell. I'd never danced properly before in my life! Actually, I tell a lie. I went to a local

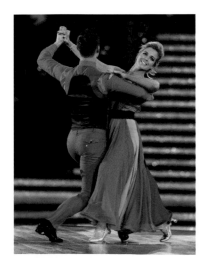

dance school when I was six or seven years old for a few months before swapping it for karate. That was the sum total of my dancing experience. It also didn't help that when my name was announced I'd get tweets saying, 'Ha! You're too big to dance' or 'Can't wait to see you try to dance in heels'. In the back of my head I was thinking, 'My mum used to call me a baby elephant... and I am rubbish in heels. What have I done?' (My friends actually got me a bracelet with a baby elephant on before the live shows and I've not taken it off since.)

I was very lucky in the partner I had, Aljaž Škorjanec. It was never a case of learning the dance and him going, 'Right – off you go!' I'd tell him I didn't feel elegant and he'd say, 'Well, you're an actress, aren't you? Act that you are.' Before each dance, he'd remind me how well I'd done in training saying, 'You've got one minute thirty seconds to prove everyone who says you're too big to dance or too muscly to be in a ballgown wrong!' We must have done, because we got to the final! During week 4 though, I tripped up the stairs as we were walking off and I think you can hear me say, 'Oh shit!' on the telly. I was like, 'I can't even walk up the frigging stairs in heels!'

Aljaž is not only an incredible dancer, but one of the funniest people I've ever met and I was having such a good time I let my diet slide, putting on nearly a stone. Everyone was like, 'You're dancing every day – how can you put weight on?' But the dancing was nothing compared to the intensity of the training I was used to and I was still getting up at 4.30am every day for the radio show, so I simply didn't prioritise food. I could have, had I really tried, but I wanted some time off, so if Aljaž and I fancied jacket potatoes with cheese, we'd have them! Whereas normally I'd think I can't really eat like I was every single day, because I was having such a laugh – and because I knew what I needed to do coming out the other end of it – it didn't bother me.

When I went back to the gym when the show was finished, I had my measurements taken. My body fat had increased, but my muscle mass had stayed the same. Evil Steve, my trainer said, 'It's fine, you just need to get back on track with your diet and carry on with your training,' and two and a half weeks later, my body was back to how it had been. Once you start training and keep at it, your body responds amazingly quickly to changes in environment. I knew mentally and physically what I had to do to get back on track, so I had no fear in letting myself relax for a bit. I can't be lean 24/7, 12 months of the year. I've got Christmasses, birthdays and all sorts I want to celebrate. I want to live! With this plan, I can. The muscle memory of someone who trains is incredible. Your body is so clever. All it wants to do is heal.

Taking chances

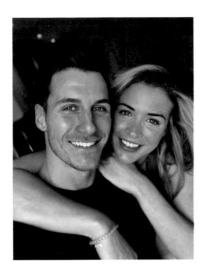

Strictly didn't just teach me to dance, break me out of my shell again and re-ignite my fondness for jacket potatoes – it also introduced me to Gorka Marquez, the man I'm now in a relationship with. One of the professional dancers on the show, Gorka and I started hanging out behind the scenes, having coffees and a laugh together. Gradually we realised we liked each other. A lot.

He's the first boyfriend I've had who truly makes me feel attractive in just a T-shirt. I've got the odd stretch mark and some cellulite on the top of my legs, like every woman, and he tells me every single day how beautiful he thinks I am. The first thing he says in the morning is, 'Good morning. I love you. How did you sleep?' I know there's time for that to stop – I'm aware we've not been together that long – but I've never had that before. And it brings this ease with it; the fact I can walk around without breathing in and I don't need to wrap a towel around me when I have just my knickers on.

We work out together – which I think has helped us to get so close. There's something incredibly supportive about someone having your back in that way, being on the same journey, wanting you to succeed and being proud of you. I talked to him about my insecurities when we had a joint PT session once. I was saying to Evil Steve, 'My cellulite's quite bad at the moment,' and Gorka jumped in and said, 'Gemma! You're a woman! You have hormones. Jesus!' It's true. Our hormones do all sorts of things to our bodies and our moods – that's our nature – but it's easy to forget that in our quest to be 'perfect'.

I post things about my life with Gorka on social media because I like the fact that other women can see I'm with someone who loves me despite me wearing no make-up in the gym and despite me not always looking pristine – it's real. Actually, wait. You know what? Just writing that made me realise that the word 'despite' is wrong! We're not good together *despite* all that, but *because* of it. Because we're open and honest and just ourselves.

Also, for the first time in my life, I am allowing myself to be vulnerable enough to be looked after by someone. Because I've always been totally independent it's a big deal for me to let a guy do anything – I can change a tyre, thank you very much, and I don't need you to pull a suitcase for me! I've struggled letting people in and showing my feelings – even down to batting off compliments as they make me uncomfortable. But letting go a little is something I'm finally allowing myself to do. It's frightening at first because I always think

'No one is perfect and looks will always fade. As long as you continue to make me laugh and make me feel secure and happy, that's all I want.'

the minute you let someone take care of you, it's harder to recover from if anything goes wrong. I think subconsciously this comes from losing my dad. I was always scared that if I allowed someone to get too close and to break down my barriers, it'd be harder to deal with if they then weren't around any more. But if you constantly put barriers up, you're always going to miss out. You're never going to give yourself the chance to experience something truly amazing. So I'm letting my guard down a bit. Plus, letting someone else pull my suitcase gives me a spare hand to hold my giant duty-free Toblerone. Winning!

By improving my self-esteem I now have a much stronger belief in my ability to cope if things go wrong. I really believe that this 12-week plan will change how people view themselves. It's given me the confidence to know my own self-worth. The physical and mental changes that happen when you do this plan truly will change your perspective on everything. You're lifting weights, you're owning it and looking after your body. Suddenly you find yourself thinking, 'I'm not going to let anybody walk over me any more. I deserve good things and good people around me'.

And, because you're doing it for yourself, you'll find you attract like-minded supportive people. People who are also secure within themselves so don't drag you down. When you feel that way, you stop comparing yourself to others. Training will help you to discover what makes you happy personally and will give you the courage and mental and physical strength to go after it.

> By improving my self-esteem I now have a much stronger belief in my ability to cope if things go wrong.

12 weeks to a whole new you

If you're reading this book, you're clearly up for making changes. For bettering yourself. For feeling the best you can be. Congratulations and hurray! That is the biggest step on this road to getting the body you love and discovering a leaner, fitter you. I feel so excited at sharing what has undoubtedly completely changed my life. It's so simple really: eat well, train well and your body and mind will thank you for it.

Whether you want a new challenge or are struggling with low self-esteem, please throw your all into this plan and I promise you'll see results that will alter how you look and feel forever. You do not have to settle for feeling sluggish, lethargic, bloated, unhealthy, overweight, insecure or bored. Feeling out of breath walking up a couple of flights of stairs isn't normal. Feeling puffed out while chasing after your kids for two minutes isn't fun. Struggling to get out of bed every single morning isn't okay. You can change those things!

Please don't do this in order to look good for someone else, for a one-off event, or to try to live up to some crappy notion of what you 'should' be. Do this to feel happier, healthier and more confident within yourself. I always think the universe doesn't give you what you want, it gives you what you need. You picked up this book for a reason, so give it your best shot.

You'll need to learn how to prep your food and not get annoyed about it – make the time, it'll be worth it (see page 48). Soon it'll just become part of your day. The other day I made myself some chicken and rice with lots of spices, put it in a Tupperware for my long train journey the next day and then, when I was on the train and the trolley packed with sweets, biscuits and sandwiches went past, I ate my pre-prepared meal instead – saving both money and that horrible bloated 'eugh' feeling that inevitably comes with eating processed foods.

This isn't about making life hard – these recipes are delicious, healthy and filling. Plus, you don't miss what you don't want!

Your body is unique. It's got you this far. Why not thank it by focusing on it for a while. Start playing for keeps rather than for instant gratification. Sometimes I still think to myself, 'My legs could be a bit slimmer, my waist, bum and hips could be a bit more J Lo. I'm quite straight up and down…' But then I catch myself, give myself a metaphorical slap, and think, 'You're 34 years old, you're half your mum, half your dad, and you've got good strong legs that have carried you everywhere you've ever been! Get over yourself.'

Make a commitment to change how you live for the next 12 weeks. Yes, it'll take some sacrifices. But is it really so awful to give up boozing and eating junk for just 12 weeks if it will utterly alter your life? 12 weeks! That's it!

Good luck!

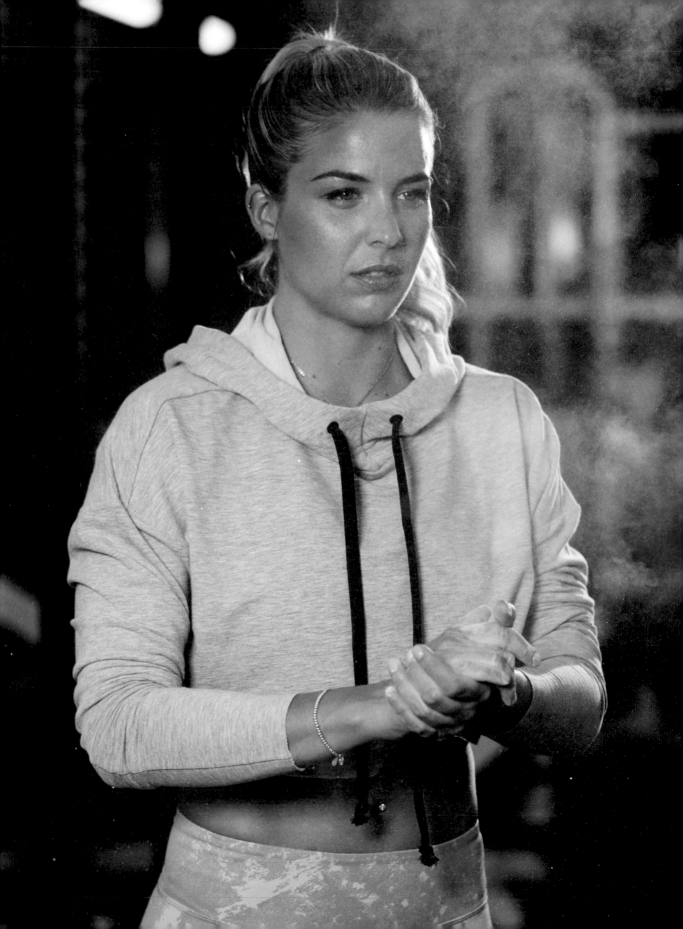

MY 10 ULTIMATE BODY PLAN COMMANDMENTS

This chapter contains the 10 commandments you need to follow to get the most out of the 12-week plan. This entire process is about feeling empowered, about making yourself accountable for your own health and wellbeing. By pledging to follow these commandments, you're promising to give this the best possible shot you can. You're vowing to take it seriously, to not throw in the towel at the first sign of trouble and to give up all faddy diets that have never and will never work. Make a commitment to change, right here and now. Take these commandments on – remember them, write them down, put your favourite as an alert on your phone to ping up during the day – and re-read them whenever you need a kick up the backside.

1 I'll remember that I don't have to be great to start, but I have to start to be great

The quote, 'You don't have to be great to start, but you have to start to be great', has pushed me to do a lot of things in my life, because we can all get held back by fear. It's easy to see yourself at the end of the journey – to picture yourself lean and healthy and loving life – but the reality of getting there can seem massively intimidating and a lot of work.

I'll be clear: this 12 weeks is going to be tough. It's going to demand sacrifice and you're going to struggle at times along the way. But there's no magic pill that'll give you these results (not even on the dark web). There should be no embarrassment associated with getting fitter. So what, you have to tell your friends you're not drinking for a while because you're on a fitness plan? So what, you're so exhausted after 10 kettlebell reps you have to lie on the floor in a puddle of your own sweat? That's bloody great! You're working hard, you're committed and you're getting stronger.

Stepping out of your comfort zone is good for you. If you never start, you'll never finish and so will never know what you can achieve. Yes, you're nervous. Yes, gyms can seem intimidating. Yes, you won't know what you're doing to start with. But you were petrified on your first day of school and you got through that. Your first kiss – you got through that. Your first day at work – you got through that. You got through all of those major things so, no matter what size or shape you are right now, you can sure as hell get through starting a fitness plan, okay?

2 I will try everything at least once and ask for help when I need it

Remember that story I told you about my mum keeping secret the fact she was taking me to the modelling agency? I've always been dismissive, uninterested or suspicious about things I don't know. When I was younger, if someone was doing something I wanted to do but was too scared to try, I'd say, 'It's not for me that, I can't be arsed with it.' When inside I'd be thinking, 'I'd love to be able to do that!' Stop talking yourself out of trying something through fear: 'I can't do that because I'm not tall enough/slim enough/funny enough/fit enough/good enough', or 'I simply don't like it'. You'll miss out on things you might actually love and that could really improve your life.

If this sounds familiar, catch yourself the next time you do it and force yourself to have a go at whatever it is you're avoiding. You might think you 'can't' do Swiss ball exercises because you'll look like a plonker, but who cares? If you don't try you'll never learn. If you're working out at home and don't get how something works, google it and watch a video or log onto an online forum and chat to others about it. Call up a friend who works out and ask them. Or bite the bullet and book a one-off personal training session. Make it work.

The same goes for food! You can't 'not like' something if you've never tried it before (just ask my mum!). And you can't dismiss certain recipes because 'I don't know how to cook'. Just try! So what, you might make a couple of mistakes. No one ever learned anything or improved themselves by being perfect first time.

3   I will fit in training (and food prep) like an important meeting

I treat training and food-prepping schedules the same way I would important meetings. I book them in and that's that. There can be a tendency to think of training as something lower down the priority scale than everything else. We often de-prioritise things we're doing for ourselves, which is silly because training is partly what gets me through the day – it's what gives me the energy to do everything else. Without it I'm sluggish, angsty and not at my best. I wouldn't be on form for the radio show first thing if I hadn't worked out or eaten well the day before.

If Becca, my agent, messages, 'When are you free for a chat?' I'll say, 'I'm training until 2pm, but after that I'm free'. Same with my friends. If we're organising a lunch, I'll say I can come after training, and it's never an issue. This is something I do that's important to me – and you need to make it important to you too. It should never be, 'Oh, it's only the gym', or 'it's only food prep' – things easily cancelled for anything else. It's essential you change your mindset about exercise, eating and looking after yourself, otherwise they'll become a drag and you'll give up. This plan shouldn't be a drag! How you prioritise it will determine what you get out of it.

Looking after yourself should be at the top of your list. We often put other people's time, comfort and schedules above our own. This is your time. This is something you're doing for you. What is more important than that? So book it in – people will get used to it, respect it and it'll save a lot of stress and guilt.

4   I will ignore my mind when it tells me to quit

It'll be your mind that wants to quit first, long before your body. That whiny little voice in your head will say, 'You're done. You're exhausted. You're not fit enough. This was a mistake. You need to stop', and so on.

I did a bungee jump once and all the way up in the cable car I was thinking, 'This is ridiculous. I won't be able to do this. I don't want to do this!' and so before I'd even got to the top I'd already talked myself out of it. Luckily someone talked me into it again, because I did do it – and bloody loved it! So much so that I went and did it again straight after because I'd enjoyed it so much.

We always doubt ourselves before we try anything new. It's a protection mechanism. But you must push past it. You CAN do this! The first three weeks are going to be the hardest. You will ache and hurt and want to gorge on chocolate, because that's safe and comforting, but I promise that if you give this your absolute all for just three weeks, you then won't want to quit. Fitting the plan into your life will have got easier (scheduling in workouts, prepping food, giving up some 'bad' habits, and letting friends and family know you're serious), plus, by that stage, you'll start seeing and believing the results. You'll already be getting leaner, fitter and healthier. You'll also feel incredibly proud of yourself for having kept at it. Your thoughts will have changed from, 'Oh God, I've got to do this workout today' to, 'Oh good, I get to do this workout today'.

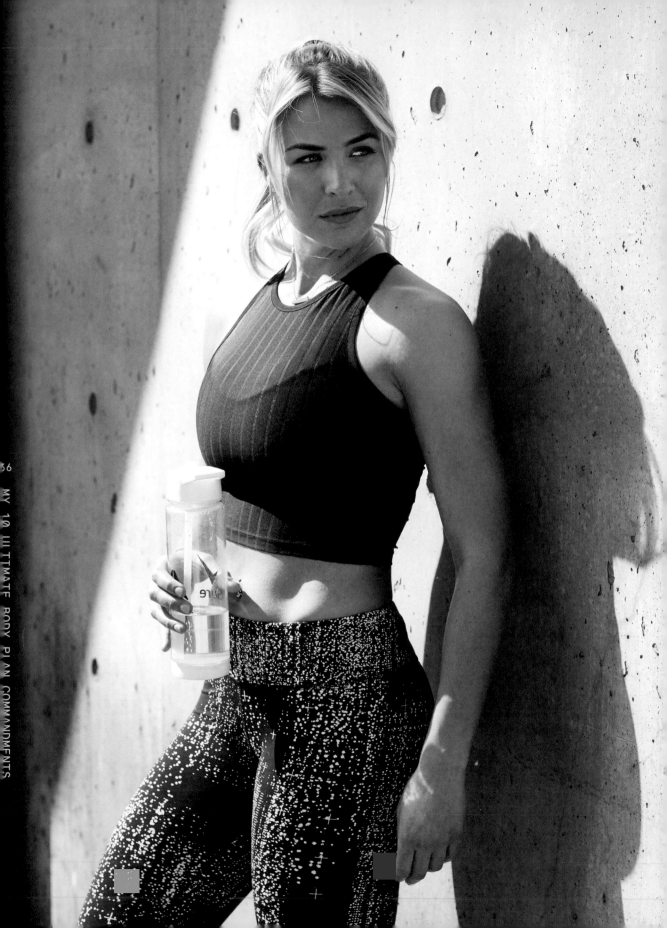

5   I will listen and pay attention to what my body is telling me

We've become experts at ignoring what our bodies are telling us, dismissing uncomfortable physical symptoms as 'normal' and just things we have to put up with. For example, feeling so bloated after lunch you have to undo the button on your jeans, or your heart racing so hard after your fifth mug of coffee that you have to sit down clutching your chest. These things aren't normal and you don't have to just 'accept' them.

We can get into habits of doing things because we 'always have'. I used to have chippy tea night every Friday. Doesn't mean I have to do that for the rest of my life – especially if I don't feel like it. Just like you don't have to drink a bottle of wine when you're with that certain mate. This plan is about becoming accountable to yourself.

What is your body telling you? Is it full? Bloated? Hungry? Thirsty? Heavy? Sluggish? What does it actually need? Is it truly craving junk or is that in your head? Start taking notice. Accept that your body will change at different stages of your cycle (there are apps that monitor mood and physicality during your period). Trust what it's telling you. If you do need to stop, don't be a hero – have a rest day. Look after yourself. If that happens once in eight or nine sessions, fine, but if it's happening once in every two or three sessions, address the reasons why. Might you be eating too much or too little? Eating the wrong things? Pushing yourself too hard? Or might it actually be your mind giving up rather than your body...?

6   I will surround myself with supportive people

Taking this step to improve yourself is a great thing and should only ever be commended. However – and I hate that I have to say this – those close to you, and perhaps even strangers, might be negative about it. I've had: 'Your body's fine, it doesn't need to change', or 'You looked better before' directed at me. People can get really annoyed when it comes to you giving up booze, feeling it somehow reflects badly on them. Fuelled by their own insecurities, they get defensive. Brush it off and stay strong.

If you're committed to this plan and to feeling your best, surround yourself with people who'll support you – and distance yourself from those who don't. Tell those closest to you what you're doing; their support will be invaluable. Even better if they'll do it with you! However, just having someone who understands that this is important to you, whether a friend or partner, will make things easier. When I was doing the 12-week programme, I'd tell my friends I'd drive because I couldn't drink, and they didn't once say, 'You're so boring! Come on!' They said, 'Great! A free taxi home!' It made all the difference.

We women need to stick together. We all know how awful it is to be brought down or made to feel like we don't measure up. The other day I saw so many women in the gym's weights section and wanted to go over and high-five them all, saying, 'It's a Sunday, you could be hung-over and lying in bed, but you look incredible!' So I did! That's what this is all about, supporting each other to be the best we can be, until eventually we change the 'Why are you doing that?' questions to 'How are you doing that?'

7 I will forgive myself when I slip up

I always say, 'We're all human. Welcome to the club.' You're going to have days when you fall off the wagon and when you feel crappy. Unless you're Hercules or a robot you're going to slip up sometimes because you're not perfect and you're not a machine.

It's very, very, rare that you'll meet someone who runs at 100% all of the time. Someone who's permanently yelling, 'I'm up for it! I'm ready!' If you slip up, shelve it and move on. There's no point dwelling on it. You can't un-eat something, you can't not-train something. It's happened, so learn from it and start again tomorrow.

It's like if you mess up an exam at school. It's done, so now what? You learn from it and do better next time. Slipping up can actually be really valuable, teaching you about patterns of behaviour. Register why you slipped – what situation or mood you were in at the time and is it likely that will happen again? For example, were you with a certain person, at a specific event or in a distinct mood? Once you know why, you can watch out for it. Maybe avoid that person while on the plan, skip those events or be more aware of yourself when you're in that mood.

But also, don't beat yourself up about it. Life wouldn't be worth living if we were always 'on' all the time. After the 12 weeks of this programme your body will know how to heal itself effectively if you do need a break in the future. You won't have to start from scratch all over again. You'll just need to up training for a bit and get back into your stride.

8 I will only compare Today-Me to Yesterday-Me, no one else

Constantly comparing yourself to others and finding yourself lacking will crush your self-esteem. A girl messaged me the other day, 'My God, you're total body goals. I wish I looked like you,' and I messaged back, 'That's a lovely thing to say, but instead of, "I want to look like you", how about, "I want to look my best"?' We always focus on our own flaws, yet see the best in other people and beat ourselves up about it.

If you find yourself constantly scrolling through social media feeds and feeling rubbish, simply stop doing it. I challenge you to try it for one day and see if you don't feel better about yourself. You wouldn't eat a food over and over again that you didn't like, so stop looking at things over and over again that you don't like! Just focus on the stuff that inspires and motivates you. Mum said once, 'If someone tells you a joke, first off it's funny. If they tell it to you again, it's quite funny. If they tell it to you again, it's boring. You don't laugh at the same thing over and over again, so why do you let the same thing hurt you over and over again?' She's very wise, my mum.

True confidence is not walking into a room, comparing yourself to everyone else and believing you're better. It's walking in, accepting everyone as they are and thinking, 'This is me. This is who I am. And I'm happy with that.' Only ever compare yourself to you from the day before. Do you feel better, healthier, stronger? If not, why not? What can you do differently today to get there?

9   I will bin my weighing scales and use positive motivators instead

I think nowadays women pay too much attention to how much they weigh and it's daft. Make a pledge to bin your scales, or at least shove them in a cupboard so you can't step on them on autopilot. Use other ways of monitoring your progress (see page 167). I used to try to inspire myself by staring at pics of other people (Kylie – I even had a pic of her as my screensaver!) – but that just made me feel bad because WE CAN NEVER LOOK LIKE ANYONE ELSE. So I would always fail in my goals. So those pics went in the bin (sorry Kylie) and instead I stuck up pictures of myself when I was at my happiest. Even if I wasn't physically where I wanted to be in those pics, seeing me so happy subconsciously drove me to strive for that feeling again.

Using those images along with my progress pictures from the plan helped me no end. The progress pics are essential, showing tangible results that'll keep you going. Also, notice how your clothes fit – are they getting looser? Do they hang better… or might a shopping spree be in order?! I would recommend you make a list of all the pros of sticking with it. Not just the general ones like 'better sleep, leaner muscles, improved wellbeing' but more personal ones. For example, 'more energy so I can play football with my kids', 'more confidence so I can start my new job feeling great', 'proving to myself I can stick to something!' You'll be surprised by how inspirational this can be and you can read over it whenever you feel in need of some motivation.

10   I shall accept that I'm stronger than I think

You may have tried exercising before and hated it. You may have tried dieting before and it didn't work. Forget all that. You're over it. This time it's different. Why? Because you're in a better headspace. First off, you know what you're aiming for this time around – a better you. Not a thinner you. Not a two-dress-sizes-lighter you. Not a you that might fit some notion of beauty you've got from social media or magazines. Ditch all that crap and instead focus on the fact you are doing this to feel healthier and stronger. The fact that you'll look totally amazing at the end of it is an added bonus.

That is why this will work. Because once you strip away those pressures and just focus on how you feel, both mentally and physically, you'll find this easy to stick to, because you'll want to. Feeling great isn't a chore.

Plus, exercise can help with low mood, stress, depression and anxiety. Often it's the last thing you feel like doing when you feel low, but force yourself to get up and do it. Just 15 minutes in, your body will release endorphins that'll lift your mood.

Believe in yourself. You can do this. You've got through all of your worst days before, haven't you? You're still here. You're reading this. That means you're stronger than you think. Remind yourself of that when you feel yourself flagging or doubt your abilities. You can stick to this and you will. You will stop punishing yourself and instead start loving yourself. Just give yourself the chance. I can't wait for you to feel fitter, leaner, stronger and happier.

let's get started!

YOUR GOALS

It's time to get real about why you want to do this 12-week plan and what completing it would mean to you. I want you to be honest with yourself. How do you want to feel, how do you want to look and why does it matter to you?

Please copy out the table opposite into a notebook you've bought specifically for this journey. I want you to fill it in now, before you start the plan. Taking the time to do this will prove you're taking it seriously and it will force you to really assess what's driving you.

Seeing your motivations written down in black and white will be inspiring, pushing you to continue when you're having a bad day (because you will have them – that's totally normal). It'll also force you to be honest with yourself. If you're doing this for someone else – because a partner has told you to or you're jealous of slimmer friends – then, if you split from your partner, or realise your friends are actually pretty miserable on their faddy diets, you'll have lost your motivation. Also, if you're doing this to fit a certain dress size by a certain date, again, once you hit that goal, where do you go from there? Filling out this table will force you to confront why you're really here. Be honest! If you are doing this for any of those reasons, write them down. Hopefully, during your journey, you'll realise your motivations have changed. I truly believe that. You'll go from, 'I want to be a size 8' to, 'I want to continue feeling bloody great!' or, 'I want to impress Dan from down the road' to, 'I want to continue impressing myself'.

In the table I also ask you to identify any potential obstacles to success. Flagging them up to yourself now – and working out ways to get around them – will take away the sting if they do come up, and you'll know what you need to do. You'll also be in a better position to try to avoid them altogether.

I'm also going to ask you to fill out another table at the end of this journey (you'll find it at the end of the book on page 234). It'll be an amazing way of seeing how far you've come and giving yourself a much deserved pat on the back.

Date today

When do you intend to start the plan?

How do you feel about starting?

What are your main objectives? (Be honest!)

How do you think you will feel physically and emotionally if you complete the 12 weeks?

What are you most looking forward to experiencing throughout the plan?

Can you list any potential stumbling blocks or obstacles you feel you might face?

How will you try to overcome these issues if they arise?

How will you reward yourself at the end of the 12 weeks?

How do you rate how you feel about yourself now, on a scale of 1 – 10, where 1 is 'I don't like myself at all' and 10 is 'I think I'm pretty damn awesome'?

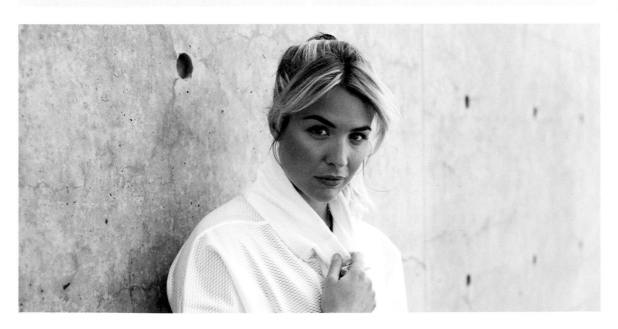

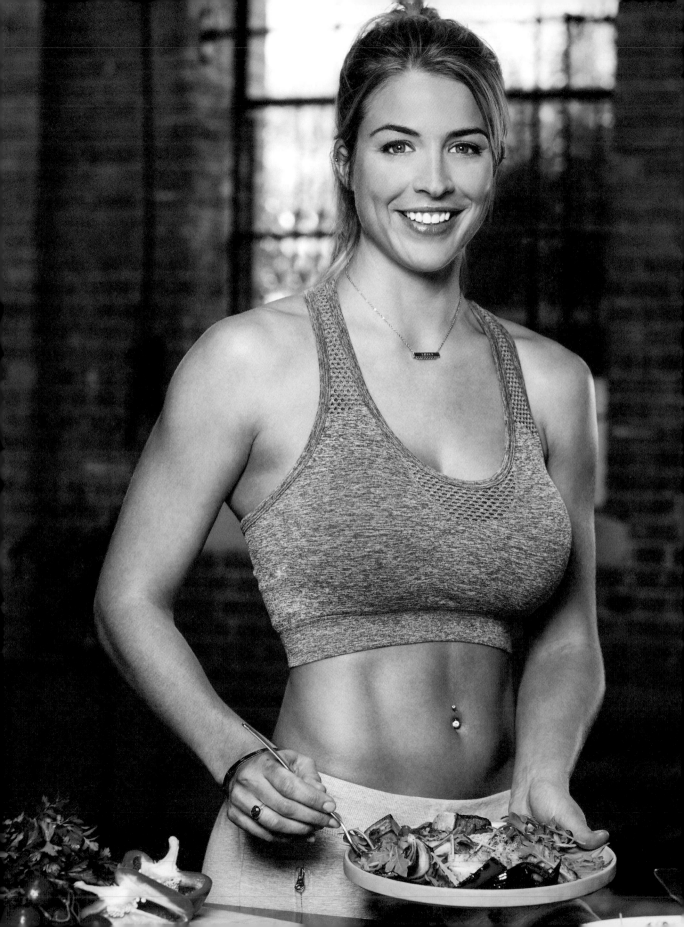

RECIPES

MAKING CALORIES WORK FOR YOU

When it comes to getting results on this plan, food is Queen. What you eat and how much you eat will determine how much fat you lose, where you lose it, how fast you lose it and whether you lose any at all. It will also determine how energetic you feel, so how inclined you are to work out, and how effective your workouts are.

Losing fat is simple: calories in versus calories out. You need to be in a calorie deficit to lose fat. If you burn more calories than you consume for an extended period of time you will gradually lose body fat. It's as simple as that, for most of us. If you have gained small amounts of body fat over the years, you are more than likely moving less and eating more – a natural process as we get older.

Lots of people advise against counting calories, however I did count calories on the 12-week plan and it worked for me, so that's what Olly Foster and I recommend you do for this plan. But, before your eyes glaze over, don't worry, it's very simple. We've calorie counted all the recipes for you so it'll be easy to work out how much you've eaten each day. All you need to know now is how many you should be eating. Please note that these are rough estimations and may need tweaking, particularly as you start losing fat. Continually track your progress and mood so you can make adjustments as and when needed.

How many calories do I need each day?
You'll need to work out two things first to get to that magic number:
1. Your BMR (basal metabolic rate)
2. Your TDEE (total daily expenditure)

Working out your BMR
Your BMR is the amount of calories you burn while doing absolutely nothing; the calories your body uses just to keep everything functioning while lying on your sofa under your dogs. To work out your BMR, you can use the calculation below, or find an online calculator. (These calculations are not 100% accurate – that would involve sophisticated equipment used in a controlled testing environment – however, they're perfect for now.)

KEY
W = Weight in kg
H = Height in cm
A = Age in years

Men	BMR = (10 x weight in kg) + (6.25 x height in cm) – (5 x age in years) + 5
Women	BMR = (10 x weight in kg) + (6.25 x height in cm) – (5 x age in years) - 161

I've filled out an example for a 30-year-old woman, who weighs 70kg and is 170cm tall. Let's call her Kate:

BMR = (10 x 70 = 700) + (6.25 x 170 = 1062) – (5 x 30 = 150) – 161
      700 + 1062 – 150 – 161 = 1451

So Kate's BMR is 1451 calories. Kate needs to consume 1451 calories per day in order to function. That's the bare minimum she needs in order to live. Any less than this and she wouldn't be able to get off the sofa (no, that isn't an option). Which brings us to working out your TDEE. This factors in how active you are; how much exercise you do, how much you move essentially.

Working out your TDEE
· BMR x 1.2 for a sedentary lifestyle with little or no exercise.
· BMR x 1.375 for light activity 1–3 days per week.
· BMR x 1.55 for moderate activity 3–5 days per week.
· BMR x 1.725 for very active 6–7 days per week.
· BMR x 1.9 for extremely active 6–7 days a week (i.e. someone with a labouring job or a professional sportsperson)

If you're participating in this programme, we're going to suggest you use the middle formula of BMR x 1.55, as chances are you already do moderate exercise.

Kate's TDEE calculation would be: TDEE is 1451 x 1.55 = 2250

This means Kate needs to consume 2250 calories per day to stay exactly the same. If she eats more, she'll gain fat; less and she'll lose fat (less than her BMR and she won't be able to function). So how much should she (and you) cut down by in order to start losing fat?

Kate's new daily calorie intake is TDEE – 500 = 1750

We reckon everyone should start by shaving 500 calories off their TDEE number as this will equate roughly to 0.5kg fat loss per week, all being well. It's a good jumping off point from which you can assess your progress, either increasing or decreasing the amount. I wouldn't recommend trying to cut down anything above 750 calories per day. That should be the absolute maximum and that's pretty steep – you might struggle to make such dramatic changes and then get dispirited. Losing body fat needs to be a gradual process for results to be long-term. However, shaving off 250 calories should be your absolute minimum aim per day. Anything less than that and you'll struggle to get off the starting blocks.

Macros. What are they and why should you care?

Olly taught me about macros when we started training together and it's essential information. It's all very well knowing what you have to do, but if you don't know *why* you're doing it, you'll be less inclined to follow through and more inclined to cheat.

Proteins, fats and carbohydrates are 'macros', or 'macronutrients' to give them their full title. Knowing about these basic food groups will help you to understand why certain meals make you feel good, bad, bloated, full, satisfied or totally uninterested.

Proteins

Protein is key for maintaining lean muscle mass. It's an essential part of every cell in the body, used to build and repair tissues, make enzymes, hormones and other chemicals and build bones, muscles, cartilage, skin, nails, hair and blood. As we don't produce protein naturally within our bodies, every bit we get must come from food.

You'll find protein in, among other things, chicken, turkey, all fish, red meat, eggs, dairy or dairy alternatives, beans, lentils and chickpeas (garbanzo beans). A lack of protein in the diet can lead to muscle loss, fatigue, irritability, decreased immunity and changes in skin pigmentation and hair texture. Lovely.

Carbohydrates

Don't believe the anti-carb hype: carbs are essential to your diet. They serve as a great energy source – at least the right carbs in the right amounts do! Yes, going low (or no) carb may help with your weight-loss goals initially and may help kick-start your plan, but long-term this is a) unsustainable and b) may even result in slowing down your metabolism, which can have the knock-on effect of messing with your menstrual cycle. Please don't avoid carbs altogether but just know what and how much to eat.

Carbs are often referred to as 'simple' or 'complex', or alternatively, 'whole' or 'refined'. Whole carbs are unprocessed and contain fibre found naturally in the food. Refined carbs have been processed so the natural fibre has been stripped out.

Examples of whole carbs include vegetables, fruit, legumes, potatoes and whole grains. Examples of refined carbs include sugar-sweetened drinks, fruit juices, pastries, white bread, white pasta and white rice. It's perhaps not surprising that we're recommending you eat whole carbs rather than refined carbs. Whole carbs are loaded with nutrients and fibre and don't cause the same spikes and dips in blood sugar levels that refined carbs do. Vegetables, fruit and whole grains are loaded with vitamins and minerals that contribute to the growth and maintenance of your muscles, while the fibre will help keep you feeling fuller for longer, control blood sugar levels and keep your digestive system running smoothly.

Fats

Fats are an essential part of your diet, helping to stabilise and regulate hormones and aiding the brain, nervous system and muscles to function. They can reduce inflammation, provide energy, protect our organs, maintain cell membranes and help the body absorb and process other nutrients. As part of a macro-balanced diet, fats help to keep us feeling fuller for longer as they are digested more slowly; they've also been proven to boost the metabolism. Examples of 'good fats' include avocados, cheese, eggs, nuts and oil.

The fats you want to avoid are 'trans fats', man-made fats that the body struggles to digest and process. They can be found in most processed foods, including doughnuts, cakes, crackers, pies and microwave meals.

Drink like a fish (literally)

I can't stress enough how important it is to stay hydrated, especially when starting a training programme to reduce body fat. We lose water through breathing, everyday sweating and going to the toilet – let alone when we're working out. The water content in the foods you eat and the drinks you drink combine to hydrate your body. If you feel thirsty you're already dehydrated!

Aim to drink around two litres of water per day. That's a solid amount to aim for, whatever your height or weight. Also, bear in mind that dehydration can also be misinterpreted as hunger, so if you feel hungry but have eaten well, drink some water to see if that curbs the temptation to snack. As for other fluid intake, avoid all fruit juices, sodas or cordials. In moderation they won't do you any harm, but nor are they doing you any good, so why bother? Try substituting a fruit juice or cordial for a herbal tea.

Alcohol

Prepare to say goodbye to alcohol, at least for a little while, during this plan. Sorry. You don't have to write it off completely – you can have a glass of wine here and there – but it's simply wasted calories. When you drink alcohol, your body uses that first as fuel for energy, delaying the fat-burning process. Also, drinking usually takes place at social occasions where snacking comes as standard – salty and fatty stuff like crisps, chips and dips. Alcohol can also make us feel more relaxed about our diets, leading not only to eating more, but eating more of the wrong stuff. Midnight kebab, anyone?

I'd be lying if I said I didn't look forward to a beer on a sunny afternoon – and you can still do that – but if you're serious about changing your body shape, please consider cutting down or laying off it totally for the duration of this plan as it really will slow down your progress. Being worried about what other people think is often a big reason why people struggle to stop drinking, and that's understandable when it's such a major part of our culture. But, like I said in the introduction, this is just 12 weeks and people will support you when they see how serious you are. If alcohol is a major part of your life, look to halve your weekly intake and take things from there. It'll ease you into telling your mates what you're doing (easier to say you're only 'having one' to start with than none at all) and the benefits you'll see and feel will inspire you to keep at it.

How flexible can you be?

Being extremely strict with food choices can be immensely boring. If you try to stick to a plan that's very limited in choice, you not only won't be getting all the nutrients you need, but you'll get bored, which means you'll be more likely to give up and, worst case scenario, you might even develop intolerances to the foods you choose to limit yourself to. So, be flexible with what you eat. Don't just pick three recipes and hammer them for weeks. Step out of your comfort zone. There are 75 recipes in this book – that's 75 opportunities to discover your new favourite dish! Feel free to adapt your own recipes to fit the plan, swapping ingredients for low-calorie versions – for example, courgetti for white pasta.

Take note of the number of servings of each recipe in this book – most serve 2, in which case the calorie information per portion will be for half of the full quantity. So if you're cooking for one, remember to halve the recipes to make sure you're getting the right amount of calories.

Yes you can have days off so you can enjoy special occasions. If you know you're going out to eat at a restaurant later on in the evening, make sure you choose a very low-cal breakfast and lunch option. How will you know how many calories are in your dinner? Chances are you won't. But don't sweat it. My rule is to always assume the worst when I'm eating out. Restaurant meals have on average 30% more calories than the same version of the meal would have if you prepared it at home. So bear that in mind and make an educated guess, or skip tracking that dinner (see tracking info opposite). Not monitoring your intake for one meal a week isn't going to affect you massively in the grand scheme of things, but eating out several times a week will. So, while doing this plan, it's worth cutting down how much you eat out.

When should I eat?

Whenever you want! Be it three meals a day with two snacks, or five mini-meals. As long as you stick to the calorie count you'll be fine. It's about learning to listen to your body. Work out how often you need to eat to feel fuller for longer.

It's all about prepping

Prepping is so important when it comes to this plan. My major bit of advice, as I mentioned in the introduction, is to put aside a couple of hours two evenings a week to bulk-cook some meals that you can then eat for lunch and dinner over the following days.

Breakfast and dinner tend to be easier to make on the spot as you're at home, so lunch is the danger zone. Be prepared. Having a Tupperware box full of healthy food you can grab on the way out will save you munching a processed sandwich during your lunch hour.

Food intolerances

Do you ever feel bloated, heavy, gassy, low on energy or get cramps a few hours after eating? That's not normal. You don't have to just put up with it. They're not just symptoms of everyday life. It means you ate something a couple of hours ago that doesn't agree with you. The number of people reporting food intolerances has risen dramatically over recent years. Some of this is down to food manufacturers trying to save money by using cheaper ingredients and some of it's down to better education about what is and isn't good for us.

If you find yourself constantly uncomfortable, start monitoring when these symptoms happen as part of your food tracking process. You can then work backwards and see what you ate before, identify what might be the culprit and try eliminating it from your diet for a while. You can also speak to your GP if things don't improve.

Tracking what you eat

Tracking how much you eat is essential for staying on course and the easiest way to do this is to use an online food tracking app, such as My Fitness Pal. Tracking is proven to improve our food choices. If you know you've actually got to write down 'pizza', 'bread and butter pudding' and 'custard', the whole meal suddenly seems a lot less appetising.

Tracking will also give you a solid basis from which to work. You'll know where and when you're slipping up and what changes you need to make to hit your targets. It will also give you a better understanding of true nutrition, portion sizes and the number of calories in certain foods. We recommend recording as you go along rather than trying to remember everything at the end of the day.

TIPS

· Don't overcook your veg as this reduces the mineral content.
· Use smaller plates. We can get into the habit of feeling we have to 'clear our plate' even if we're full halfway through a meal. Using smaller plates will help you to manage your portions.
· Take time over your meal. By eating more slowly you're giving your body time to properly digest – and time to register when you're full. We eat so quickly nowadays we're already on thirds before realising the button on our jeans has popped.

 VEGAN

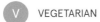 VEGETARIAN

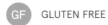 GLUTEN FREE

 VARIATIONS

I have included variations in some recipes, but do be aware that changing the ingredients in a dish will alter the calorie count. If an ingredient is listed as 'optional', it is not included in the calorie counts.

BREAK-FASTS

Breakfast Bars

330kcals PER BAR | ⑪ MAKES 12 | ⏱ PREP TIME 15 MIN | 🍲 COOKING TIME 30-35 MIN

These bars are perfect for breakfast on-the-go or as a power snack during the day. They're so easy to make and will stay fresh for up to five days in an airtight container.

300g (10oz/3¼ cups) rolled oats

75g (3oz/scant ¾ cup) chopped pecans, walnuts or hazelnuts

100g (4oz/scant ¾ cup) chopped ready-to-eat dried apricots

100g (4oz/generous ½ cup) chopped stoned (pitted) dates

50g (2oz/generous ½ cup) dried cranberries or blueberries

50g (2oz/scant ½ cup) raisins

4 tbsp mixed seeds, e.g. pumpkin, sunflower, sesame, chia, hemp, linseeds

150g (5oz/generous ½ cup) butter, plus extra for greasing

6 tbsp runny honey

a few drops of vanilla extract

1. Preheat the oven to 170°C/150°C fan/325°F/gas 3. Lightly butter a 30 x 20cm (12 x 8in) baking tin (pan) and line with parchment paper.

2. Put the oats, nuts, dried fruits and seeds in a large bowl.

3. Heat the butter and honey in a small saucepan set over a low heat, stirring until the butter melts. Stir into the oat mixture with the vanilla extract and mix well. If it's too dry, add some more melted butter; if it's not firm enough and too sticky, add some more oats.

4. Transfer to the prepared tin and smooth the top, pressing down firmly with the back of a metal spoon to level the surface. Bake in the oven for 30–35 minutes until crisp and golden brown.

5. Remove and leave to cool slightly before cutting into 12 bars. Leave in the tin until completely cold, then remove and store in an airtight container.

💡 TIP: Try toasting the whole nuts in a dry frying pan (skillet) for 2 minutes to bring out their aroma and flavour before cooling and chopping. Delicious!

Crunchy Granola with Fruit

PER SERVING: 415kcals | ⚟ SERVES 4 | ⏱ PREP TIME 10 MIN | 🍲 COOKING TIME 20-25 MIN

This recipe makes four servings of granola, but you can double the quantities and make a bigger batch as it'll keep well in an airtight container for a couple of weeks. There are no hard and fast rules about what you put in, so feel free to use whatever you've got to hand: walnuts, pecans, almonds, chopped dates, dried cranberries etc., but note that this will affect the calorie count per serving. I like to serve it with yoghurt, sliced banana, stewed rhubarb or any seasonal fruits.

2 tbsp coconut oil

2 tbsp maple syrup

100g (4oz/1¼ cups) rolled oats

40g (1½oz/scant ¼ cup) roughly chopped hazelnuts

25g (1oz/scant ¼ cup) sunflower seeds

25g (1oz/scant ¼ cup) pumpkin seeds

2 tbsp sesame seeds

50g (2oz/scant ½ cup) raisins

½ tsp ground cinnamon

200g/7oz strawberries or raspberries

200g (7oz/scant 1 cup) 0% fat Greek yoghurt

runny honey, for drizzling (optional)

1. Preheat the oven to 170°C/150°C fan/325°F/gas 3. Line a large baking tray (cookie sheet) with parchment paper.

2. Heat the coconut oil and maple syrup in a saucepan set over a low heat. When the coconut oil melts, stir in the oats, nuts, seeds, raisins and cinnamon. Make sure that everything is well coated.

3. Spread the mixture out in a thin layer on the lined baking tray and bake in the oven for 15–20 minutes, stirring once or twice, until golden brown and crisp. Leave to cool before transferring to an airtight container.

4. Serve the granola with the berries and yoghurt, drizzled with honey, if using.

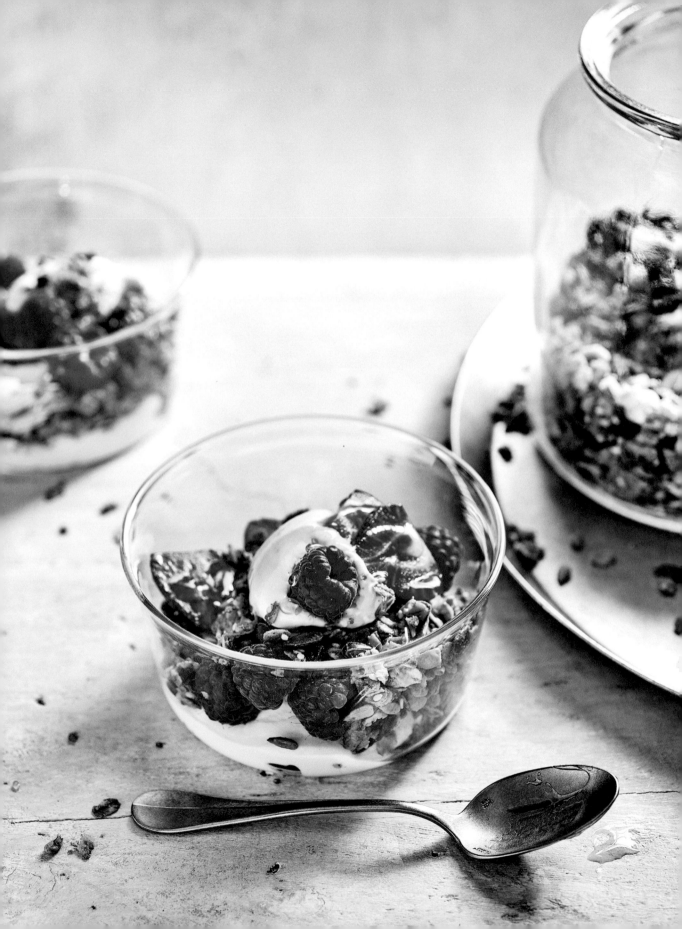

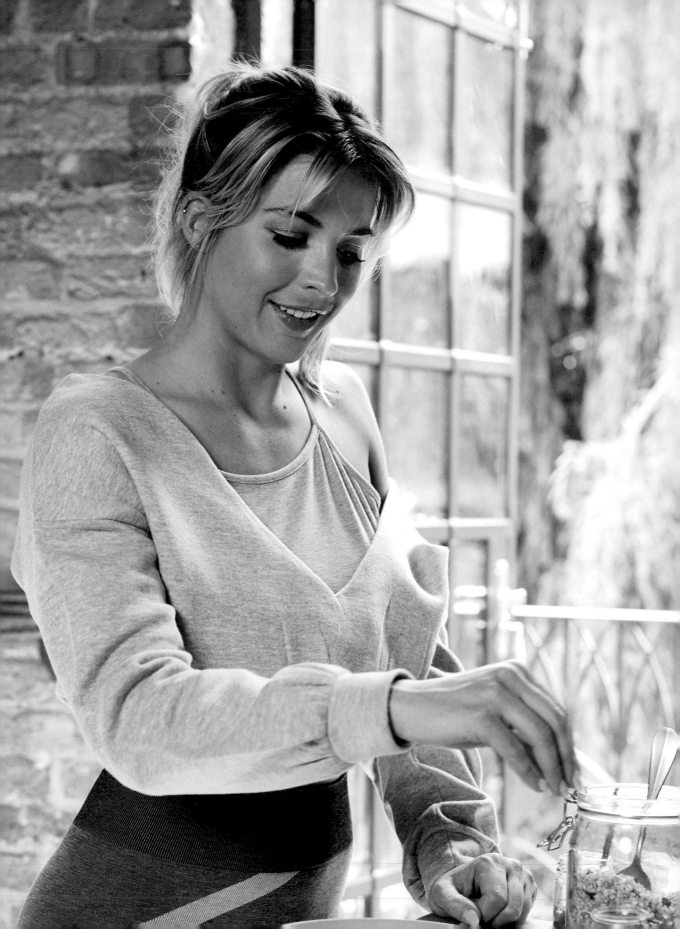

Overnight Oat & Yoghurt Pots

215kcals PER SERVING | ￦ SERVES 2 | ⏱ PREP TIME 10 MIN | ❄ CHILL TIME OVERNIGHT

This is so easy – you just assemble the little pots the evening before and chill them in the fridge overnight so the yoghurt and milk get to work their magic and the oats swell up. If you choose to use full-fat Greek yoghurt instead of 0% fat yoghurt, each pot will be 275kcals.

250g (9oz/generous 1 cup) 0% fat
   Greek yoghurt
60ml (2fl oz/4 tbsp) unsweetened
   almond milk
4 tbsp rolled oats
1 tbsp mixed seeds, e.g. pumpkin,
   sunflower, chia, flax seeds
200g/7oz mixed berries, e.g.
   strawberries, raspberries,
   blueberries
1 banana

1. In a bowl, mix together most of the Greek yoghurt with the milk, oats and seeds.
2. Divide the mixture between two wide-neck glass jars or clear containers. Add a layer of berries then cover them with the remaining yoghurt. Top with the rest of the berries.
3. Cover the jars or containers and chill in the fridge overnight. The following morning, slice the banana, divide it between the pots and eat for breakfast.

💡 VARIATIONS:

· Drizzle with some runny honey.
· Add a few drops of vanilla or almond extract to the yoghurt mixture.
· Stir in the grated zest of 1 orange before chilling.
· Sprinkle with chopped hazelnuts or walnuts before serving.

Peanut Butter Porridge

390kcals PER SERVING | 🍴 SERVES 2 | ⏱ PREP TIME 5 MIN | 🍲 COOKING TIME 10 MIN

Porridge is always a healthy and warming way to start the day, and because it's high in fibre and low GI it makes you feel full, so you're less likely to feel hungry and need a snack mid-morning.

85g (3oz/1 cup) rolled oats
240ml (8fl oz/1 cup) water
240ml (8fl oz/1 cup) unsweetened
   almond milk
a pinch of salt
2 tbsp peanut butter (no added
   sugar)
2 tsp maple syrup

TOPPING
1 small banana, sliced
2 tbsp toasted pecans or almonds,
   chopped
maple syrup, for drizzling

1. Put the oats, water, almond milk and salt in a non-stick saucepan and set over a low heat. Stir gently with a wooden spoon until the oats start to soften, then increase the heat and bring to the boil, stirring constantly.

2. Reduce the heat to a low simmer and cook gently for 2–3 minutes until all the liquid has been absorbed and the porridge is thick and creamy.

3. Remove the pan from the heat and stir in the peanut butter and maple syrup.

4. Spoon the porridge into two breakfast bowls and top with the sliced banana and nuts. Serve hot, drizzled with maple syrup.

💡 VARIATIONS:

· Stir in some dark (bittersweet) chocolate chips just before serving.
· Swap the peanut butter for another nut butter, such as almond or cashew.
· Top with fresh berries or cacao nibs.

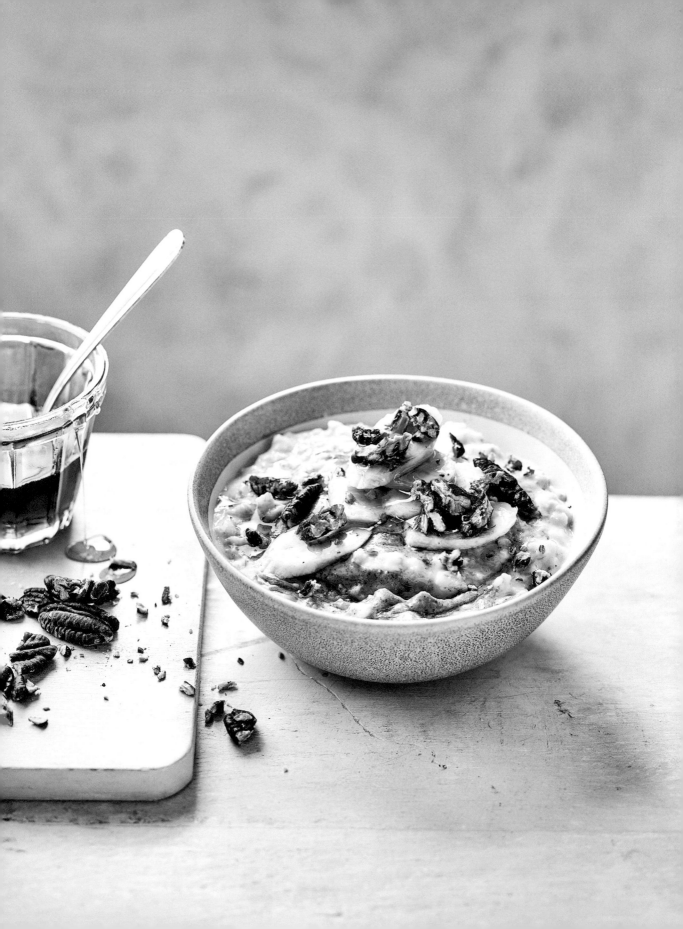

Baked Greek Eggs

390kcals PER SERVING | SERVES 2 | PREP TIME 10 MIN | COOKING TIME 15 MIN

This dish is a breakfast showstopper. One of those meals you can't believe is healthy because it's so filling (and good-looking!), but it's full of calcium and tastes incredible.

100ml (3½fl oz/scant ½ cup) full-fat milk

2 tbsp 0% fat Greek yoghurt

juice of ½ small lemon

100g/4oz spinach, washed, trimmed and shredded

6 medium free-range eggs

80g/3oz feta cheese, diced

40g/1½oz stoned (pitted) black olives

2 tbsp chopped dill or parsley

salt and freshly ground black pepper

1. Preheat the oven to 200°C/180°C fan/400°F/gas 6.
2. Mix together the milk, yoghurt and lemon juice in a jug and season lightly with salt and pepper.
3. Cover the bottom of a large shallow ovenproof dish with the spinach. Pour the milk mixture over the top. Make six indentations in the spinach and carefully crack an egg into each one. Dot the top with the feta and olives, then sprinkle with the herbs.
4. Bake in the oven for about 15 minutes until the spinach is tender and the egg whites are set but the yolks are still runny.

TIP: If you don't have any feta, sprinkle some grated Cheddar over the top instead, before baking.

Bacon & Egg Muffins

150kcals PER SERVING | MAKES 6 | PREP TIME 10 MIN | COOKING TIME 20–25 MIN

High in protein and low in carbs, these savoury muffins are simple to make and delicious.

12 extra-thin rashers (slices) lean back bacon

3 medium free-range eggs

200g/7oz courgettes (zucchini), grated

30g (1oz/generous ¼ cup) Parmesan cheese, grated

freshly ground black pepper

1. Preheat the oven to 180°C/160°C fan/350°F/gas 4.
2. Line 6 muffin tin (pan) holes with overlapping bacon rashers to make little bacon 'cups'. Press down lightly to seal any gaps so the filling can't leak out.
3. Beat the eggs with some black pepper in a bowl and mix in the grated courgettes (zucchini) and Parmesan. Spoon the mixture carefully into the bacon cups.
4. Bake in the oven for 20–25 minutes until the bacon is crisp and the egg filling is golden brown and has set.
5. Eat hot or cold.

Green Breakfast Smoothie

262kcals PER SERVING | ⦙⦙⦙ SERVES 1 | ⏱ PREP TIME 10 MIN

This green smoothie is packed with nutrients, vegetable fibre and protein, meaning you'll feel full until lunch.

25g/1oz kale, washed and trimmed

25g/1oz spinach, washed and trimmed

25g (1oz/2 tbsp) chocolate protein powder

10g/⅓oz whole raw almonds

1 tbsp chia seeds

1 tbsp flax seeds

400ml (14fl oz/1½ cups) unsweetened almond milk

3 ice cubes

1. Put all the ingredients in a blender and blitz until smooth.

2. Pour into a tall glass and drink immediately.

💡 **VARIATION:**

· Swap the chocolate protein powder for vanilla-flavoured protein powder.

Asparagus Dippy Eggs

335kcals PER SERVING | ⦙⦙⦙ SERVES 2 | ⏱ PREP TIME 10 MIN | 🍲 COOKING TIME 10 MIN

Full of antioxidants, asparagus is incredibly healthy and makes a great alternative to traditional bread 'soldiers'.

4 medium free-range eggs

olive oil spray

200g/7oz asparagus spears, trimmed

juice of ½ small lemon

140g/5oz thinly sliced lean Parma ham

salt and freshly ground black pepper

PER SERVING: 335kcals

1. Carefully lower the eggs into a saucepan of simmering water and cook gently for 5–7 minutes – 5 minutes for a very runny yolk, 7 for an almost set yolk. Remove and place in egg cups.

2. Meanwhile, spray a griddle pan with oil and set over a medium heat. Add the asparagus and cook for 8–10 minutes, turning occasionally, until tender and just starting to char (but still firm).

3. Season the asparagus and sprinkle with a little lemon juice before rolling up each spear in a slice of Parma ham.

4. Cut the tops off the eggs and serve with the asparagus dippers and salt and pepper.

Egg & Mushroom Cups

405kcals PER SERVING | ⟊⟊⟊ SERVES 2 | ⏱ PREP TIME 10 MIN | 🍲 COOKING TIME 20 MIN

These stuffed mushrooms topped with fried eggs are great for a healthy weekend brunch. Kale is a key ingredient as it's a powerhouse of nutrients, especially vitamins A, B6, C and K, as well as calcium and magnesium.

4 large flat portobello or field mushrooms
1 tsp coconut oil
¼ small red onion, diced
1 small red (bell) pepper, deseeded and diced
60g/2oz kale, trimmed and finely chopped
½ tsp sweet paprika
45g (1½oz/scant ½ cup) Cheddar cheese, grated
1 tbsp vegetable or olive oil, plus extra for spraying
4 medium free-range eggs
a pinch of cayenne, for sprinkling
salt and freshly ground black pepper

1. Preheat the oven to 190°C/170°C fan/375°F/gas 5.
2. Remove the stalks from the mushrooms and chop them finely. Set aside. Place the mushroom 'cups' on a baking tray (cookie sheet). Season them with salt and pepper and spray lightly with oil. Bake in the oven for 15 minutes until tender.
3. Meanwhile, heat the coconut oil in a wok or large frying pan (skillet) set over a medium-high heat. Add the onion and stir-fry for 3–4 minutes until it starts to soften. Add the diced mushroom stalks, red (bell) pepper, kale and paprika and cook for 5–6 minutes, stirring occasionally, until all the vegetables are tender. If the mixture is too dry, add a splash of water to moisten it. Stir in the grated cheese.
4. Divide the mixture between the baked mushrooms and return to the oven for 5 minutes until the cheese melts.
5. Meanwhile, heat the oil in a clean frying pan and fry the eggs until the whites are set. Remove and drain on kitchen paper (paper towels).
6. Serve the hot mushroom cups topped with the fried eggs sprinkled with cayenne.

BREAKFASTS

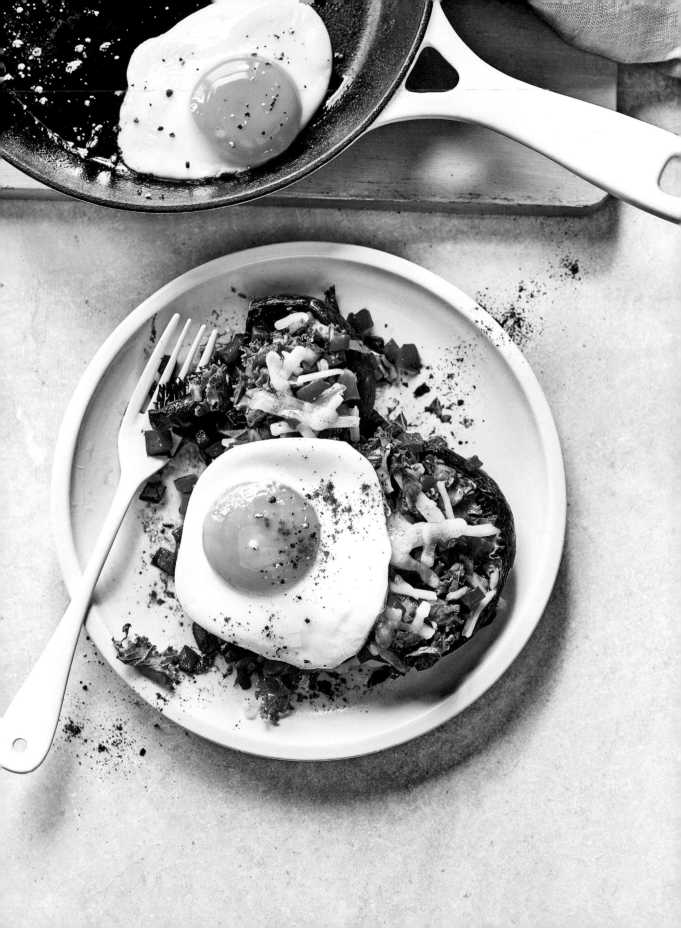

Green French Toast

345kcals PER SERVING | ⫻ SERVES 2 | ⏱ PREP TIME 5-10 MIN | 🍲 COOKING TIME 4-6 MIN

I love this savoury French toast. It's so easy to make and is great for a weekend brunch. Sometimes I serve it with sliced banana and some soft cheese instead of tomatoes.

2 medium free-range eggs

3 tbsp semi-skimmed milk, nut milk or soya milk

a handful of herbs, e.g. parsley, chives, basil, coriander (cilantro), finely chopped

2 spring onions (scallions), trimmed and finely chopped

2 medium slices of multi-seed or wholegrain bread

1 tbsp olive oil, plus extra for brushing

200g/7oz cherry tomatoes on the vine

2 tbsp maple syrup or runny honey

salt and freshly ground black pepper

1. Beat the eggs and milk together in a shallow bowl. Stir in the herbs and spring onions (scallions), then season with salt and pepper.

2. Put the slices of bread into the beaten egg mixture and leave to soak for 2–3 minutes, turning them over halfway through, so all the beaten egg is absorbed.

3. Heat the oil in a large non-stick frying pan (skillet) set over a low–medium heat. When it's really hot, carefully add the soaked bread and cook for 2–3 minutes until crisp and golden brown underneath. Turn them over and cook the other side.

4. Meanwhile, cook the tomatoes in an oiled griddle pan set over a medium–high heat until slightly softened (yet still holding their shape) and charred.

5. Serve the French toast, drizzled with the maple syrup or honey, topped with the tomatoes.

 VARIATIONS:

· Sprinkle the French toast with paprika or drizzle it with your favourite hot sauce.

· If you like it spicy, add some diced green chilli to the beaten eggs before soaking the bread.

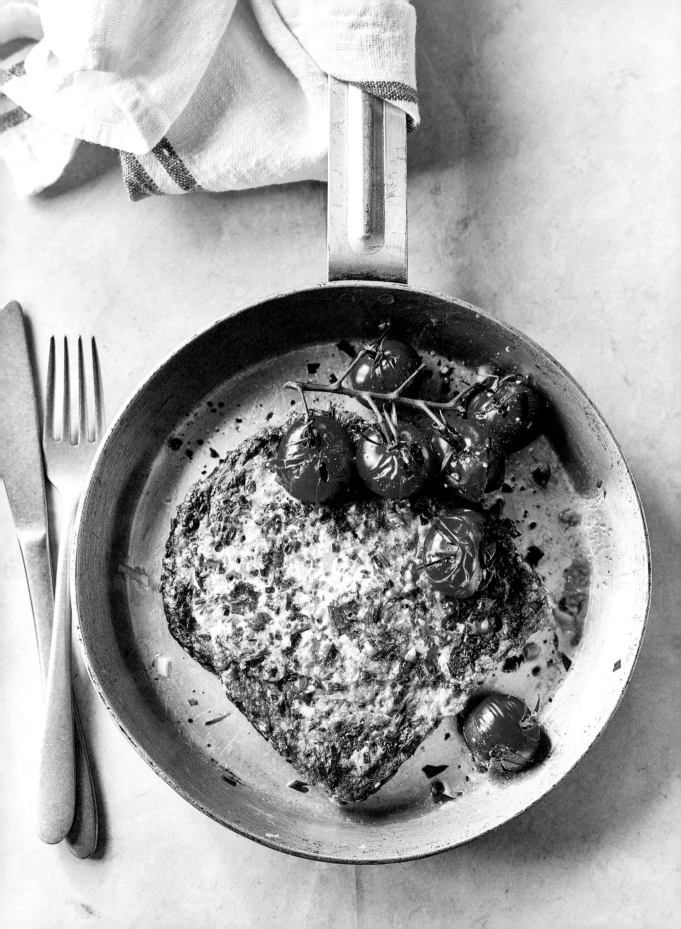

Eggs with Broccoli & Sun-dried Tomatoes

329kcals PER SERVING | SERVES 2 | PREP TIME 5 MIN | COOKING TIME 8–10 MIN

People shy away from eating veg at breakfast – don't! Broccoli and eggs are a great combo, especially as the broccoli will give you a good hit of vitamin C.

100g/4oz broccoli florets, cut into
   bite-sized pieces
6 medium free-range eggs
2 tsp butter
60g/2oz sun-dried tomatoes,
   chopped
salt and freshly ground black pepper

1. Steam the broccoli florets for 4–5 minutes until tender but not mushy.
2. Beat the eggs in a bowl with some salt and pepper. Melt the butter in a non-stick frying pan (skillet) set over a medium heat, then pour in the beaten eggs and cook, stirring occasionally with a wooden spoon, for 2 minutes.
3. Add the broccoli and sun-dried tomatoes and cook, stirring gently, for about 2 minutes until the mixture scrambles and just sets (avoid overcooking the eggs or they will be rubbery). Serve immediately.

VARIATION:

- Try adding snipped chives, cooked diced mushrooms or chopped spring onions (scallions).

Courgette Ribbons with Smoked Salmon

283kcals PER SERVING | SERVES 2 | PREP TIME 5 MIN | COOKING TIME 3–4 MIN

Protein-rich cottage cheese, teamed up here with smoked salmon, is a great alternative to eggs.

200g/7oz courgettes (zucchini)
1 tsp vegetable or coconut oil
100g (4oz/½ cup) natural cottage cheese
200g/7oz thinly sliced smoked
   salmon or salmon trimmings, cut
   into strips
salt and freshly ground black pepper
lemon wedges, for squeezing

1. Using a potato peeler, cut the courgettes (zucchini) lengthways into thin ribbons.
2. Heat the oil in a frying pan (skillet) set over a medium–high heat and add the courgette ribbons. Cook for 3–4 minutes, turning them occasionally, until they are just tender but still retain some bite. Season lightly with salt and pepper.
3. Divide the courgettes between two serving plates and top with the cottage cheese and smoked salmon. Grind a little black pepper over the salmon and serve immediately with lemon wedges for squeezing.

Green Veggie Breakfast Fritters

290kcals PER SERVING | ⊞ SERVES 2 | ⏱ PREP TIME 15 MIN | 🍲 COOKING TIME 12 MIN

These little fritters are so simple to make and taste amazing when they're served piping hot from the pan. Make them for a weekend breakfast or brunch and serve with grilled tomatoes or mushrooms.

2 medium free-range eggs

2 tbsp grated Parmesan cheese

200g/7oz courgettes (zucchini), grated

75g/3oz baby leaf spinach, roughly chopped

3 spring onions (scallions), trimmed and finely chopped

a small bunch of parsley, mint or dill, finely chopped, plus extra for sprinkling

grated zest of 1 lemon

25g (1oz/¼ cup) plain (all-purpose) flour

1 tbsp olive oil

100g (4oz/scant ½ cup) 0% fat Greek yoghurt

salt and freshly ground black pepper

Ⓥ

1. Preheat the oven to 110°C/90°C fan/225°F/gas ¼.

2. Beat the eggs in a large bowl and stir in the Parmesan, vegetables, herbs and lemon zest. Gently stir in the flour and season with salt and pepper.

3. Heat the oil in a non-stick frying pan (skillet) set over a medium–high heat. When the pan is hot, add a few heaped dessertspoons of the batter, one at a time, so they have room around them to spread out.

4. Cook the fritters for about 2 minutes until golden brown and set underneath, then flip them over and cook the other side for a further minute or two. Remove from the pan and place on a warm plate lined with kitchen paper (paper towels). Pop into the oven to keep warm while you cook the remaining fritters in the same way, adding more oil to the pan if necessary.

5. Serve the warm fritters with Greek yoghurt sprinkled with herbs.

💡 VARIATIONS:

· Add some canned sweetcorn kernels or grated carrot to the fritter mixture.

· Instead of Parmesan, add grated Cheddar cheese or even some crumbled feta cheese.

Smoked Salmon & Avocado Scrambled Eggs

375kcals PER SERVING | ⏲ SERVES 2 | ⏱ PREP TIME 10 MIN | 🍲 COOKING TIME 4–5 MIN

Eggs and salmon are a healthy breakfast combo made in heaven. They both pack a protein punch, and the nutrient-dense salmon is an excellent source of vitamins, minerals and essential omega-3 fatty acids, which contribute to a healthy brain, heart and joints.

6 medium free-range eggs

2 tsp butter

1 small ripe avocado, peeled, stoned (pitted) and diced

100g/4oz smoked salmon, chopped

a few sprigs of parsley or chives, finely chopped

salt and freshly ground black pepper

lemon wedges, to serve

1. Beat the eggs in a bowl with a little salt and pepper.
2. Melt the butter in a non-stick saucepan set over a medium–high heat. Pour in the beaten eggs and cook, stirring with a wooden spoon, for 2–3 minutes.
3. Add the avocado, smoked salmon and parsley or chives and continue stirring for about 1 minute until the eggs are scrambled and set, and everything is warmed through.
4. Remove from the heat immediately and divide the scrambled eggs between two warm serving plates. Serve with wedges of lemon.

💡 VARIATIONS:

· Add some chopped spring onion (scallion) or a little diced chilli to the scrambled eggs.
· Serve the eggs on a slice of multi-seed or wholegrain toast.

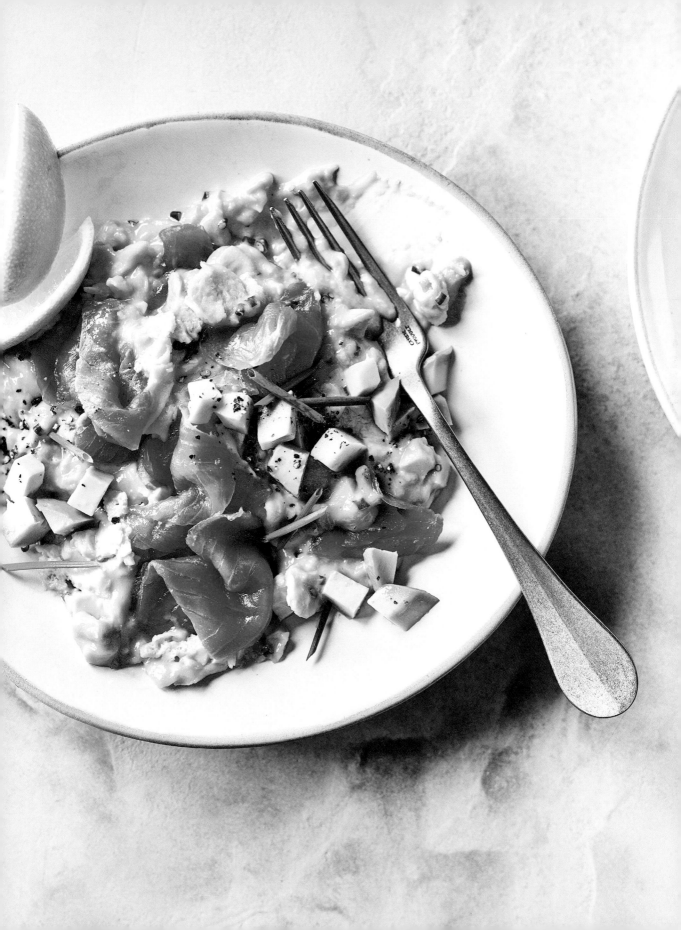

Vegetable Frittata

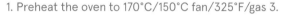 337kcals PER SERVING | SERVES 2 | PREP TIME 10 MIN | COOKING TIME 25–35 MIN

This is a great way to get a load of vegetables into your first meal of the day. You can even make the frittata the night before and eat it cold for breakfast, or take some to work as a healthy packed lunch.

100g/4oz asparagus spears, trimmed
    and cut into small chunks
1 small red (bell) pepper, deseeded
    and cut into small chunks
2 tsp olive oil
150g/5oz courgette (zucchini),
    grated
6 medium free-range eggs, beaten
a handful of parsley, finely chopped
40g/1½oz feta cheese, diced
salt and freshly ground black pepper

1. Preheat the oven to 170°C/150°C fan/325°F/gas 3.
2. Put the asparagus and red (bell) pepper on a baking tray (cookie sheet) and drizzle with 1 teaspoon of the oil. Season lightly with salt and pepper and roast in the oven for 10–15 minutes until the vegetables are starting to soften and crisp up.
3. Heat the remaining oil in a non-stick frying pan (skillet) with a heatproof handle (not wood as it's going to be put into the oven). Add the courgette (zucchini) and cook over a medium heat for 4–5 minutes, stirring occasionally, then stir in the baked asparagus and red pepper.
4. Stir in the beaten eggs, parsley, feta and a little seasoning and cook for 3–5 minutes until the bottom of the frittata is set and golden brown.
5. Place the pan in the oven and cook for 5–10 minutes until the top is set and golden brown and the frittata is cooked.
6. Remove from the oven to cool a little before sliding the frittata out of the pan onto a board. Cut into wedges and serve lukewarm.

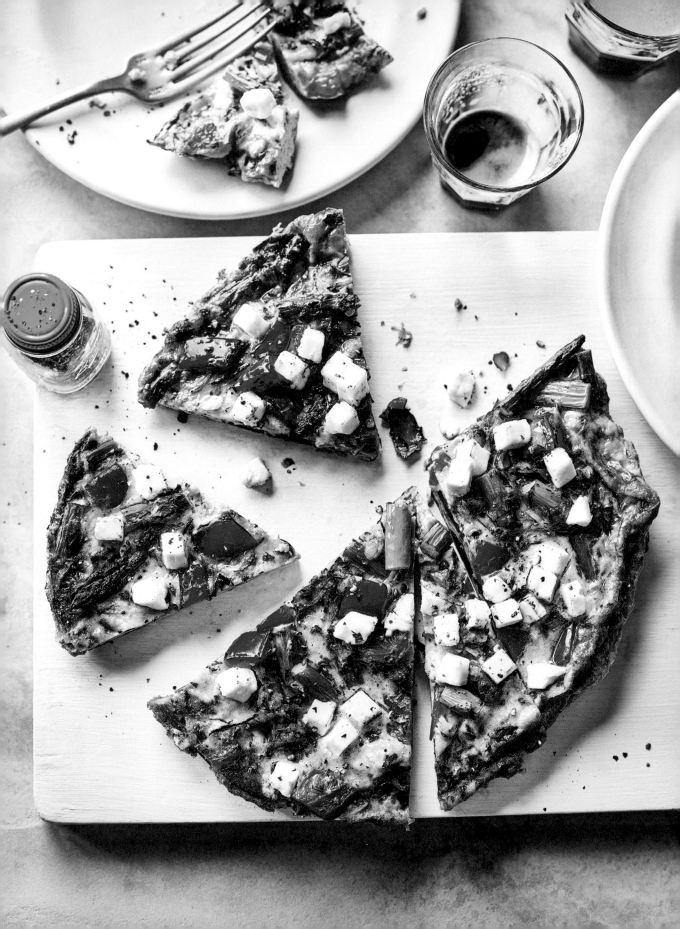

Mexican Breakfast Burritos

338kcals PER SERVING | ⑪ SERVES 2 | ⏱ PREP TIME 10 MIN | 🍲 COOKING TIME 8–10 MIN

Wraps are very versatile and make a great breakfast, lunch or snack. I sometimes drizzle these with hot sauce or serve them with guacamole.

olive oil spray

4 spring onions (scallions), trimmed and chopped

1 small red chilli, deseeded and diced

200g (7oz/1 cup) canned refried beans

a handful of coriander (cilantro), chopped

2 large wholewheat tortillas or wraps

a handful of crisp lettuce, e.g. cos (romaine) or iceberg, shredded

4 tbsp hot salsa

4 tbsp grated Cheddar cheese

salt and freshly ground black pepper

2 tbsp 0% fat Greek yoghurt, to serve

hot sauce, for drizzling (optional)

1. Lightly spray a non-stick frying pan (skillet) with oil and set over a low–medium heat. Cook the spring onions (scallions) and chilli for 3 minutes until softened. Add the refried beans together with a good splash of water. Stir well and heat through gently – the mixture shouldn't be too thick as you'll need to spread it over the tortillas. Add the coriander (cilantro) and season to taste with salt and pepper.

2. Meanwhile, warm the tortillas or wraps in the oven or on a griddle pan set over a low heat.

3. Spread the refried bean mixture over the warm tortillas or wraps and top with the shredded lettuce, salsa and cheese.

4. Roll up the tortillas or fold the ends in to enclose the filling and then roll. Serve immediately with the Greek yoghurt.

💡 VARIATION:

· Instead of refried beans, scramble some eggs with the spring onions, chilli and herbs. Assemble the burritos in the same way. Delicious!

BREAKFASTS

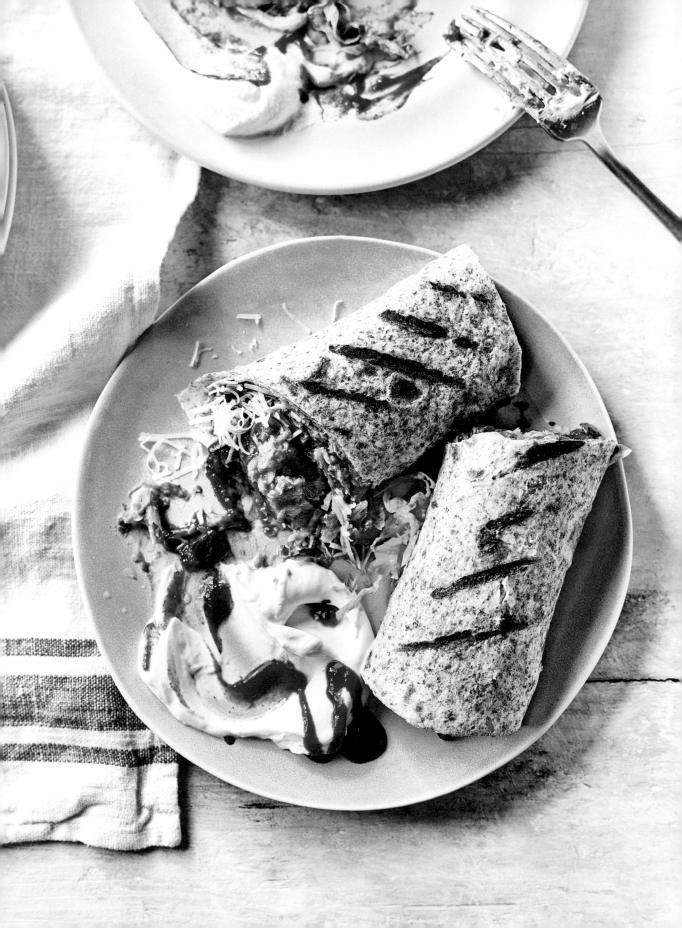

Herring & Avocado Salad

468kcals PER SERVING | ▟▙▜ SERVES 2 | ⏱ PREP TIME 10 MIN | 🍲 COOKING TIME 4–5 MIN

We often follow 'rules' when it comes to meals, only eating certain things at certain times. Well, if you've never had fish or salad for breakfast before, it's time to start now. Whack some herrings on a fresh salad and start your day right. It's a game-changer.

75g/3oz kale, washed and trimmed

100g/4oz cucumber, sliced

50g/2oz cooked beetroot (beets), diced (not in vinegar)

40g/1½oz radishes, sliced

1 small ripe avocado, peeled, stoned (pitted) and diced

25g/1oz stoned (pitted) black olives,

275g/10oz rollmop herrings

lemon wedges, for squeezing

DRESSING

juice of ½ lemon

1 tbsp olive oil

1 tbsp grated Parmesan cheese

1 tsp wholegrain mustard

a dash of water

1. Make the dressing by whisking all the ingredients together in a bowl.

2. Steam the kale for 4–5 minutes until just tender. Pat dry with kitchen paper (paper towels).

3. Put the kale in a bowl with the other vegetables, avocado and black olives. Toss gently in the dressing.

4. Divide between two serving plates and top with the rollmop herrings. Serve with wedges of lemon for squeezing over the herrings.

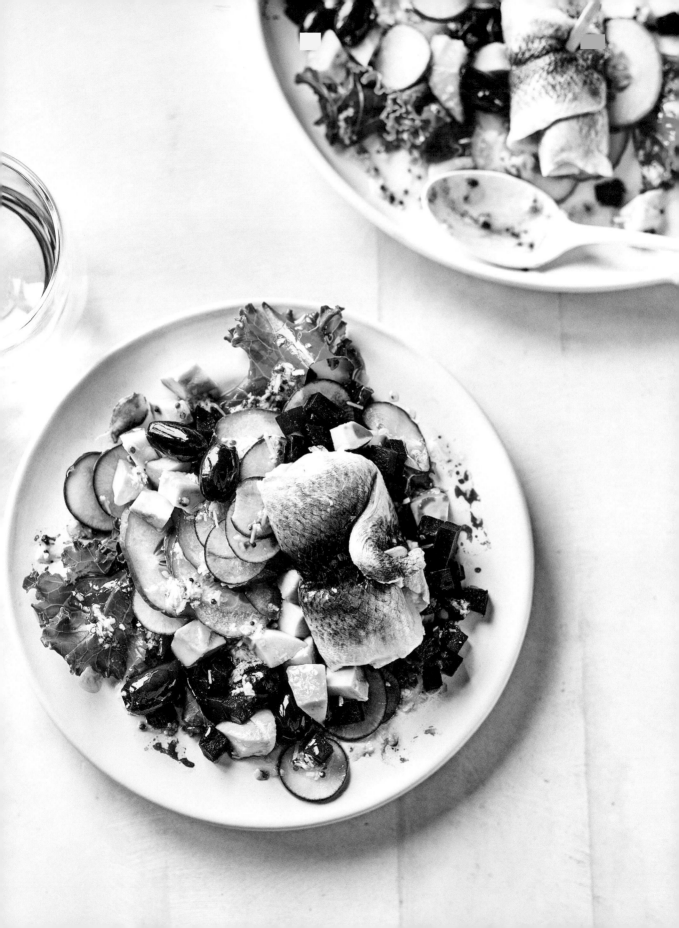

SNACKS

Spicy Parmesan Roasted Cashews

270kcals PER SERVING | ¶¶¶ SERVES 8 | ⏱ PREP TIME 5 MIN | 🍲 COOKING TIME 8-10 MIN

I love cashews – they're delicious and packed with vegetable protein, vitamin B6, essential minerals and healthy monounsaturated fat. Whole blanched almonds can also be roasted like this if you want to mix things up a bit.

1 tbsp vegetable oil
3 tbsp runny honey
3 tbsp finely grated Parmesan cheese
1 tsp sweet paprika
a pinch of cayenne
300g (10oz/2 cups) unsalted cashews
1 tsp fine sea salt crystals

1. Preheat the oven to 190°C/170°C fan/375°F/gas 5. Line a baking tray (cookie sheet) with a raised edge with parchment paper.
2. Whisk the oil and honey together in a bowl, then whisk in the Parmesan, paprika and cayenne. Toss the cashews in this mixture.
3. Spread the cashews out in a single layer on the lined baking tray and sprinkle with the sea salt. Bake in the oven for 8–10 minutes, turning the nuts halfway through, until they are golden brown and fragrant. Check on the nuts frequently to make sure they don't catch and burn.
4. Leave to cool on the baking tray – they will become more crispy as they cool. Store in an airtight container for up to a week.

💡 VARIATIONS:

· Add some garlic powder, finely chopped rosemary or oregano, ground cumin, allspice, chilli powder, smoked paprika or black pepper.
· Instead of using oil and honey, make a healthier, lower-calorie version with a beaten egg white. Add the cheese and spices as above and cook in the same way.

Spicy Roasted Chickpeas

115kcals PER 50g / 2oz SERVING | ▮▮▮ MAKES 500g | ⏱ PREP TIME 10 MIN | 🍲 COOKING TIME 25–35 MIN

Snacks can be some of the best meals of the day. These crunchy roasted chickpeas taste so good, you'll think they are bad for you, but trust me they're not. These will stay fresh and crisp for a few days (if you can avoid munching them for that long!).

2 x 400g (14oz/3 cups) cans
   chickpeas (garbanzo beans),
   rinsed and drained
2 tbsp olive oil
½ tsp fine sea salt
1 tsp chilli powder
1 tsp ground cumin
1 tsp smoked paprika
a good pinch of cayenne pepper

1. Preheat the oven to 200°C/180°C fan/400°F/gas 6.
2. Put the drained chickpeas (garbanzo beans) in a bowl with the olive oil, sea salt and ground spices. Toss lightly together until they are evenly coated.
3. Spread them out in a single layer on a baking tray (cookie sheet) with a raised edge. Roast in the oven for 25–35 minutes, turning them once or twice, until crisp and golden brown.
4. Leave to cool on the baking tray, then serve or store in a sealed container or a plastic bag at room temperature.

🔅 VARIATIONS:

· To make Thai-spiced chickpeas, swap the spices above for a pinch of dried chilli flakes, ½ teaspoon Thai curry paste, ½ teaspoon ground turmeric and 1 tablespoon nam pla (Thai fish sauce).
· To make Greek-spiced chickpeas, swap the spices above for 1 teaspoon ground coriander seeds, 1 teaspoon ground fennel seeds, ½ teaspoon ground cumin seeds, 1 teaspoon garlic powder and the juice of ½ small lemon.

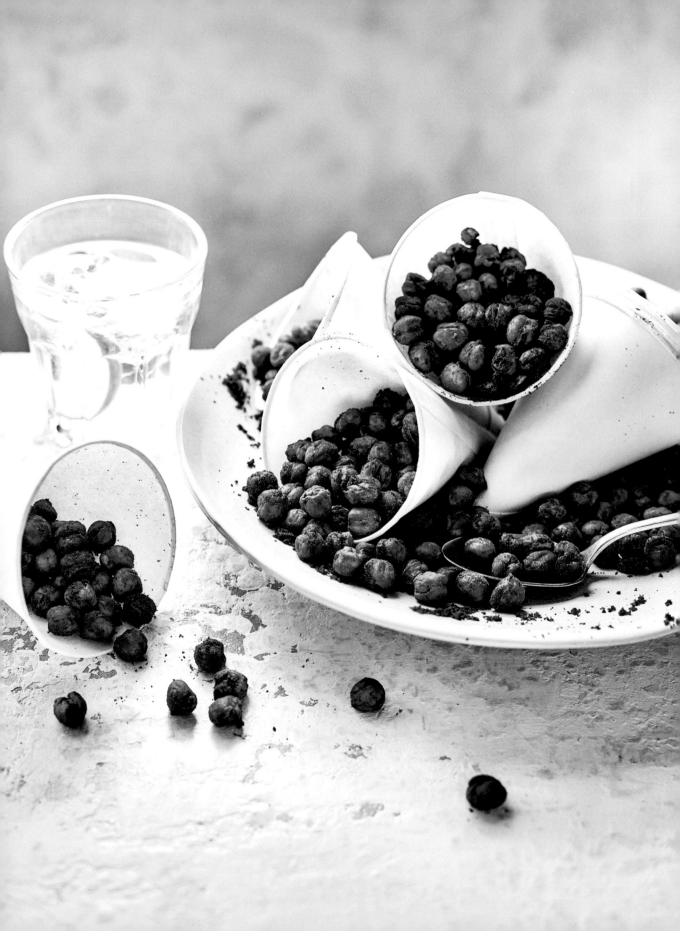

Santorini Fava Dip

290kcals PER SERVING | ¶¶¶ SERVES 8 | ⏱ PREP TIME 10 MIN | 🍲 COOKING TIME 1 HR 10 MIN

This brilliant purée made with split peas comes from the romantic Greek island of Santorini, but is eaten all over Greece. It's perfect for vegetarians and vegans wanting to boost their protein and dietary fibre intake. Serve it as a dip for warm pitta bread or raw vegetables or as an accompaniment to grilled halloumi, chicken or fish. It will keep in an airtight container in the fridge for up to 4 days.

450g (1lb/2 cups) yellow split peas
   (dry weight)
1 small onion, quartered
2 garlic cloves
1 bay leaf
a few sprigs of thyme
100ml (3½fl oz/scant ½ cup) fruity
   green olive oil, plus extra for
   drizzling
juice of 1 lemon
salt and freshly ground black pepper
¼ red onion, diced, to serve
2 tbsp whole capers, rinsed, to serve

1. Rinse the split peas in a sieve under cold running water. Put them in a large saucepan with the onion, garlic and herbs. Cover with plenty of cold water and bring to the boil. Skim off any foamy scum that forms on the surface.
2. Lower the heat and simmer gently for about 1 hour or until the split peas are very soft and most of the water is absorbed. Drain in a sieve suspended over a bowl to catch the cooking liquid. Discard the onion and herbs but keep the garlic.
3. Tip the split peas and garlic into a blender or food processor. With the motor running, start adding the olive oil through the feed tube in a steady stream. Add the lemon juice and blitz again. If the fava dip is thick and stiff rather than light, thin it with some of the reserved cooking liquid. Alternatively, you can mash the fava roughly with a potato masher if you like a more chunky texture. Season to taste with salt and pepper.
4. Put the fava dip in a bowl and drizzle with olive oil. Serve it lukewarm or cold, sprinkled with the red onion and capers.

💡 VARIATION:

· Try sprinkling the fava dip with diced spring onions (scallions), chilli, preserved caper leaves or a dusting of paprika or cayenne. Drizzle with lemon juice.

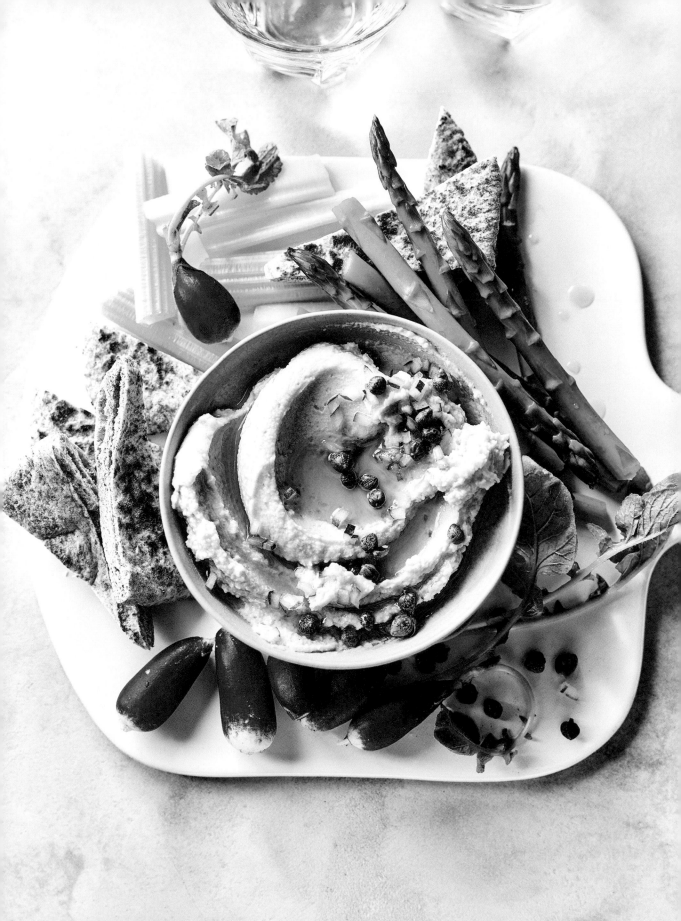

Quick Green Hummus

260kcals PER SERVING | ¶¶¶ SERVES 8 | ⏲ PREP TIME 15 MIN

Homemade hummus absolutely wipes the floor with shop-bought stuff. Make up a batch to keep in the fridge for a quick snack when you're feeling peckish or your blood sugar levels are low. Spread it over low-GI oatcakes (50kcals per oatcake) and boost your energy levels.

2 x 400g (14oz/3 cups) cans
   chickpeas (garbanzo beans),
   rinsed and drained
3 tbsp tahini
3 garlic cloves
a large bunch of basil
juice of 1 large lemon
100ml (3½fl oz/scant ½ cup) fruity
   green olive oil, plus extra for
   drizzling
a pinch of sea salt crystals
sweet paprika, for dusting
oatcakes, to serve (optional)

1. Put most of the chickpeas (garbanzo beans) in a blender or food processor (reserve a few for the garnish) with the tahini, garlic, basil leaves and lemon juice and blitz.
2. With the motor running, add the olive oil through the feed tube in a thin, steady stream until you have a relatively smooth paste. If it's too thick for your liking, thin it with 1 tablespoon hot water, more lemon juice or some of the chickpea can liquid. It should be quite soft (but not runny) and a little grainy, not too smooth. Season to taste with the sea salt.
3. Transfer the hummus to a bowl and drizzle with olive oil. Scatter with the reserved whole chickpeas, dust with paprika and serve with oatcakes. Store in an airtight container in the fridge for up to 4 days (if it lasts that long).

░̣ VARIATIONS:
· Swap the basil for parsley, mint or coriander (cilantro).
· Sprinkle the hummus with toasted seeds.
· Stir in 1 tablespoon 0% fat Greek yoghurt for a creamier texture.

Chia Seed Pudding

245kcals PER SERVING | SERVES 2 | PREP TIME 10 MIN | CHILL TIME OVERNIGHT

Chia seeds are packed with nutrients and omega-3 fatty acids and make a delicious porridge-like pudding or snack.

30g/1oz peeled piece of ripe avocado
1 tsp almond butter
60g (2oz/4 tbsp) chocolate or vanilla protein powder
200ml (7fl oz/generous ¾ cup) unsweetened almond milk
4 tbsp chia seeds

1. Put the avocado, almond butter, protein powder and almond milk in a blender and blitz until smooth.
2. Pour into a large bowl and stir in the chia seeds, distributing them throughout the mixture. Cover with cling film (plastic wrap) and chill in the fridge overnight.
3. The next day, divide the mixture between two bowls, or transfer to airtight containers or glass-lidded jars to take to work with you.

 VARIATION:
· Serve the chia pudding topped with fresh berries or sliced fruit (peaches, bananas or mango).

Nut Butter Banana Toasties

310kcals PER SERVING | SERVES 2 | PREP TIME 5 MIN

I like to use crunchy peanut butter to make these toasties but any nut butter works well. If you have a toasted sandwich maker, you can make them with two slices of bread per person (an extra slice of bread will add 70kcals to each serving).

2 medium slices of wholegrain or multi-seed bread
2 tbsp peanut, almond or cashew butter
1 medium banana, mashed or thinly sliced
30g/1oz plain (bittersweet) chocolate, grated

1. Toast the bread lightly and spread it with the nut butter right up to the edges.
2. Top with the mashed or sliced banana and sprinkle with the grated chocolate. If you like, pop the toasties under a hot grill (broiler) briefly to melt the chocolate.

 VARIATION:
· Use toasted wholemeal muffins or bagels instead of wholegrain or multi-seed bread.

Sticky Nutty Flapjacks

320kcals PER SERVING | ††† MAKES 12 | ⏱ PREP TIME 10 MIN | 🍲 COOKING TIME 20 MIN

Everybody loves flapjacks, but instead of using the traditional butter, sugar and golden syrup, these ones are made with dates, peanut butter and maple syrup.

100g (4oz/½ cup) stoned (pitted) dates

¾ tsp bicarbonate of soda (baking soda)

150g (5oz/generous ½ cup) smooth peanut butter (no added sugar)

2 egg whites

120ml (4fl oz/½ cup) maple syrup

400g (14oz/4 cups) rolled oats

100g (4oz/1 cup) chopped hazelnuts

1 tsp ground cinnamon

a few drops of vanilla extract

1. Preheat the oven to 180°C/160°C fan/350°F/gas 4. Line a 30 x 20cm (12 x 8in) baking tin (pan) with parchment paper.

2. Put the dates and bicarbonate of soda in a heatproof bowl and cover with boiling water. Leave to soak for 10 minutes or so until softened, then drain the dates, reserving the soaking water.

3. Put the dates in a blender or food processor with the peanut butter, egg whites and maple syrup and blitz until smooth.

4. Transfer the mixture to a bowl and add the oats, hazelnuts, cinnamon and vanilla extract. Stir until well combined and sticky. If it's too dry, add a little of the reserved date soaking liquid; if it's too wet, add some more oats.

5. Spoon the mixture into the prepared tin and press it down with a metal spoon or spatula to level the top. Bake in the oven for about 20 minutes or until golden brown.

6. Remove from the oven and leave to cool in the tin before cutting into 12 squares. Store in an airtight container for up to 5 days.

 VARIATION:

· Use runny honey instead of maple syrup.

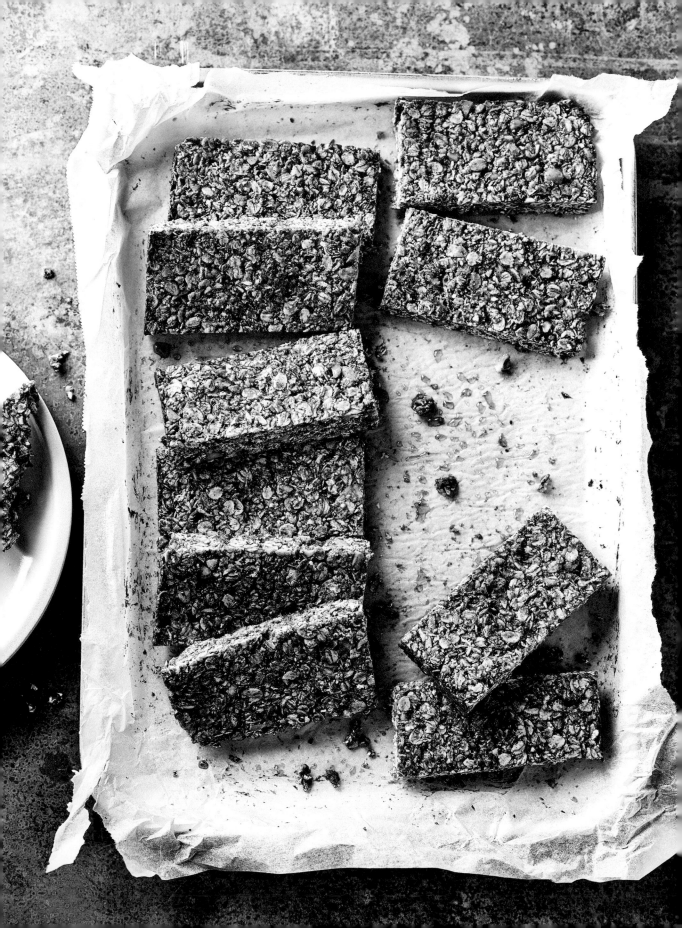

Frozen Banana Choc Lollies

175kcals PER SERVING | ▐▐▐ MAKES 8 | ⏱ PREP TIME 15 MIN | ❄ FREEZE TIME 10-11 HRS

These amazing lollies are a healthier version of a good old-fashioned choc ice and are a great way of using up leftover ripe bananas that nobody wants to eat! You will need eight wooden lolly sticks.

4 ripe bananas

100g (4oz/generous ½ cup) dark (bittersweet) chocolate chips

½ tsp coconut oil

75g (3oz/scant ½ cup) chopped unsalted nuts, e.g. walnuts, almonds, hazelnuts, peanuts, cashews

1. Peel the bananas and cut them in half horizontally (not lengthways). Insert a lolly stick into the sliced ends and place them side by side on a baking tray (cookie sheet) lined with parchment paper. Freeze for at least 10 hours.

2. When you're ready to make the lollies, melt the chocolate chips and coconut oil in the microwave on medium heat in 20-second bursts or in a heatproof bowl suspended over a pan of gently simmering water. When they are melted and glossy, remove from the heat immediately.

3. Holding the end of the stick, dip a frozen banana into the melted chocolate and then roll it in the chopped nuts. Repeat with the remaining bananas and place them back on the lined tray. Return to the freezer for at least 30 minutes until the chocolate is set. They will keep in the freezer for up to 1 week.

💡 **TIP:** Try toasting the whole nuts in a dry frying pan (skillet) for 2 minutes to bring out their aroma and flavour before cooling and chopping. Delicious!

SNACKS

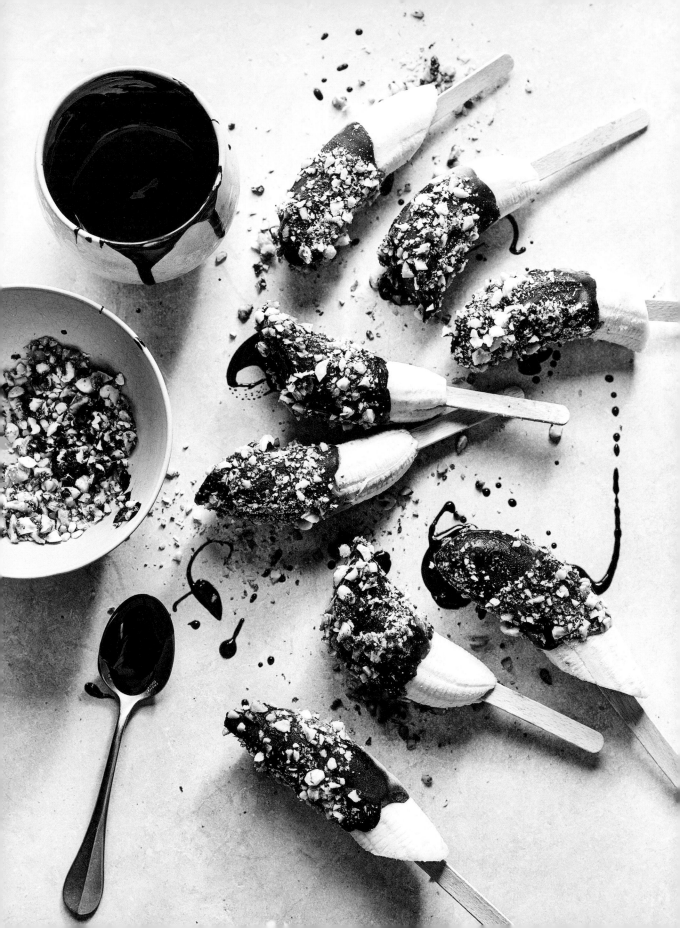

Chocolate Coconut Energy Bites

105kcals PER BITE | ▮▮▮ MAKES 18 BITES | ⏱ PREP TIME 15 MIN | ❄ CHILL TIME 30 MIN

These little energy balls are a great pick-me-up as they're full of essential minerals and vitamins. They also freeze well for up to 3 months, so I recommend making a huge batch.

250g (9oz/1½ cups) soft Medjool dates, stoned (pitted) and chopped

60g (2oz/scant ¾ cup) shredded unsweetened coconut

60g (2oz/½ cup) chopped walnuts

2 tbsp peanut or almond butter

2 tbsp unsweetened cocoa powder

1 tbsp chia or flax seeds

1 tbsp coconut oil

a pinch of sea salt

1. Put the dates in a food processor and blitz until you have a sticky paste.
2. Add half of the shredded coconut together with the walnuts, nut butter, cocoa powder, seeds, coconut oil and salt. Blitz again until everything is well combined, adding 1–2 tablespoons cold water to moisten the mixture if it's too dry.
3. Take small pieces of the mixture and shape each one into a small ball (approximately 2cm/1in diameter) – you should get 18 balls in total – then roll them in the remaining coconut. Place on a baking tray (cookie sheet) lined with parchment paper and chill in the fridge for at least 30 minutes to firm up.
4. Store the balls in an airtight container in the fridge for up to 7 days, or in the freezer for up to 3 months (defrost at room temperature before eating).

💡 VARIATIONS:

· For an intensely chocolaty flavour, try adding a handful of dark (bittersweet) chocolate chips to the mixture after blitzing, before rolling into balls.
· Use chopped almonds, hazelnuts or pecans instead of walnuts.
· Add some cacao nibs or vanilla extract before blitzing.

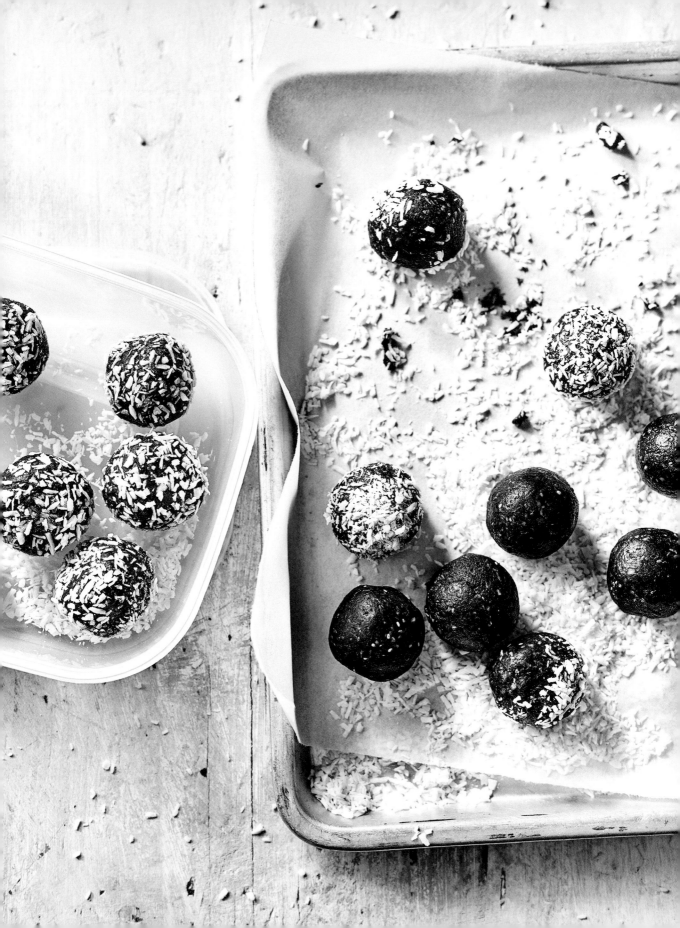

LIGHT MEALS & LUNCHES

Spinach & Sweet Potato Tortilla

440kcals PER SERVING | ||| SERVES 2 | ⏱ PREP TIME 15 MIN | 🍲 COOKING TIME 25-30 MIN

Tortillas are incredibly satisfying to both cook and eat. They look great, they taste even better, they're easy to share and you can graze on them throughout the day. They also work hot or cold, making them perfect for a packed lunch or picnic.

300g/10oz sweet potato, peeled and cubed

1 tbsp olive oil

1 onion, chopped

1 red (bell) pepper, deseeded and chopped

2 garlic cloves, crushed

1 red chilli, deseeded and diced

100g/4oz spinach, washed, trimmed and shredded

4 medium free-range eggs

1 tbsp grated Parmesan cheese

salt and freshly ground black pepper

1. Cook the sweet potato in a saucepan of lightly salted boiling water for about 5 minutes until it's just tender but still holds its shape. Drain well.

2. Heat the oil in a non-stick frying pan (skillet) set over a low-medium heat, add the onion, red (bell) pepper and garlic and cook, stirring occasionally, for 6-8 minutes until softened but not browned. Add the chilli, drained sweet potato and spinach and cook for 3-4 minutes, stirring once or twice, until the spinach wilts.

3. Beat the eggs in a bowl and season lightly with salt and pepper. Pour into the frying pan and reduce the heat. Cook gently for 5-6 minutes until the tortilla is set and golden brown underneath. Preheat the grill (broiler).

4. Sprinkle with grated cheese and pop the pan under the preheated grill for about 5 minutes until the top is lightly browned and the tortilla is set.

5. Slide the cooked tortilla out of the pan onto a wooden board and let it cool a little. When it's lukewarm, cut into wedges and serve (or chill for another meal).

-💡- **VARIATION:**

· Use pumpkin or butternut squash instead of sweet potato.

LIGHT MEALS & LUNCHES

BBQ Chicken & Roasted Sweet Potato Salad

470kcals PER SERVING | ▐▐▐ SERVES 2 | ⏱ PREP TIME 15 MIN | 🍲 COOKING TIME 25-30 MIN

You can barbecue the chicken and roast the vegetables the evening before, chill them in the fridge overnight and then toss in the dressing the following morning, ready to pop into a lunchbox to take to work.

300g/10oz sweet potato, peeled and cut into chunks

1 red onion, cut into small wedges

1 large red (bell) pepper, deseeded and cut into strips

2 tbsp olive oil

1 tsp coriander seeds

2 tsp cumin seeds

2 x 100g/4oz skinned chicken breasts

1 small bag of salad leaves, e.g. rocket (arugula), watercress, baby spinach

salt and freshly ground black pepper

HONEY LEMON DRESSING

1 garlic clove, crushed

1 tsp peeled and grated fresh ginger root

2 tsp honey mustard

1 tbsp cider vinegar

juice of 1 lemon

2 tbsp cold water

1 tsp poppy seeds

1. Preheat the oven to 200°C/180°C fan/400°F/gas 6 and prepare the barbecue (if using).

2. Put the sweet potato, onion and red (bell) pepper in a roasting pan and drizzle with the olive oil. Coarsely grind the coriander and cumin seeds with an electric spice grinder or pestle and mortar, then sprinkle them over the vegetables. Season lightly with salt and pepper. Roast in the oven for 25–30 minutes, turning the vegetables once or twice, until just tender and golden brown.

3. Meanwhile, cook the chicken over hot coals on the barbecue, turning it once or twice, for about 15 minutes until golden brown and cooked right through. Alternatively, cook in an oiled hot griddle pan. Remove from the heat and slice.

4. Whisk all the dressing ingredients together in a bowl, shake in a screw-top jar or blitz in a blender until well blended and smooth.

5. Put the roasted vegetables and salad leaves in a bowl and toss lightly with half of the the dressing. Divide between two serving plates and arrange the sliced chicken on top. Drizzle with the reserved dressing.

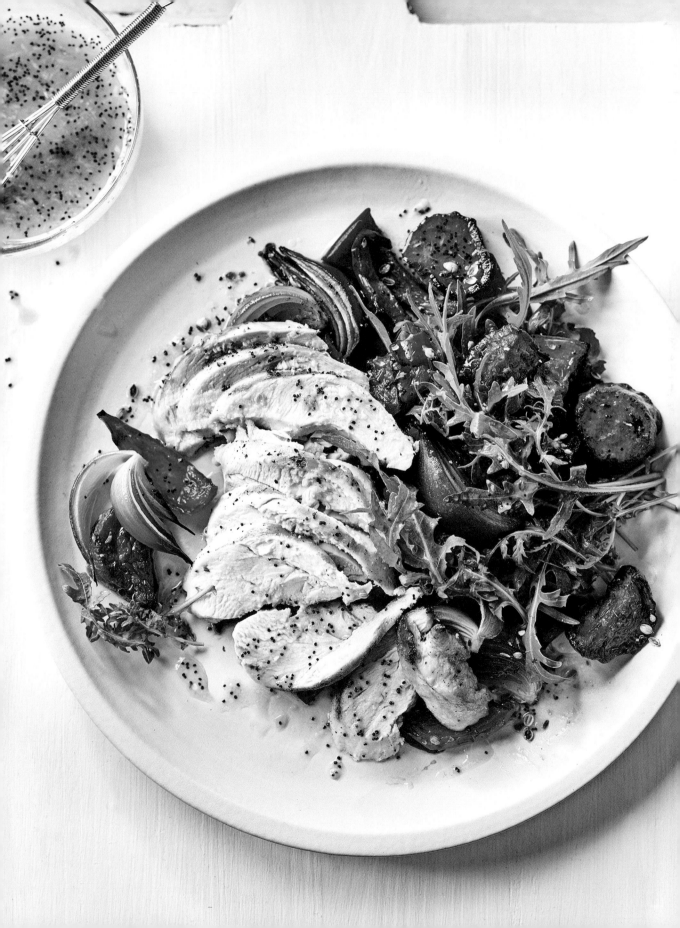

Beetroot & Couscous Lunchbox Salad

450kcals PER SERVING | ₩₩₩ SERVES 2 | ⏱ PREP TIME 10 MIN | 🍲 SOAK TIME 10 MIN

This summery salad will brighten up any day (we should put more fruit in salad, I've decided). You can boil or roast the beetroot yourself or buy a packet of ready-cooked beetroot in the supermarket (just make sure it doesn't come in vinegar). The mango and orange combine to give this a lovely fresh kick.

100g (4oz/generous ½ cup) couscous (dry weight)

150ml (5fl oz/scant ¾ cup) boiling chicken or vegetable stock

1 tbsp olive oil

juice of 1 orange

a handful of parsley, leaves chopped

a handful of mint, leaves chopped

250g/9oz cooked and peeled beetroot (beets), cut into chunks (not in vinegar)

4 spring onions (scallions), trimmed and chopped

1 small mango, peeled, stoned (pitted) and cubed

60g/2oz feta cheese, diced

salt and freshly ground black pepper

1. Put the couscous in a heatproof bowl and pour the boiling stock over it. Stir well, cover with cling film (plastic wrap) and leave for about 10 minutes or until the couscous swells and all the liquid is absorbed.

2. Remove the cling film, fluff up the couscous with a fork and stir in the olive oil, orange juice and herbs. Season to taste with salt and pepper.

3. Stir in the beetroot (beets), spring onions (scallions) and mango, then crumble the feta cheese over the top. Cool and transfer to sealed containers for a packed lunch or eat straight away.

💡 VARIATIONS:

· Try this with roasted carrots, butternut squash or pumpkin.

· Use papaya instead of mango.

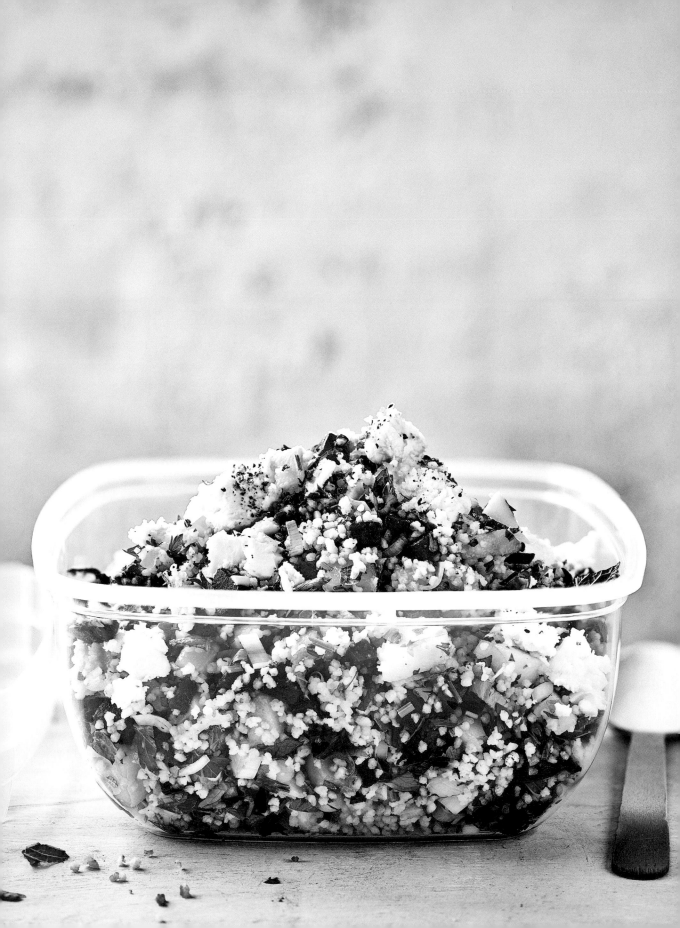

Salade Niçoise Pittas

420kcals PER SERVING | ⅲ SERVES 2 | ⏱ PREP TIME 15 MIN | 🍲 COOKING TIME 8 MIN

A classic salade niçoise with a twist – bung it in some pitta! This super-healthy lunch will fill you up until dinner, guaranteed.

50g/2oz fine green beans, trimmed

2 medium free-range eggs

1 x 160g/5oz can tuna in spring water, drained

2 spring onions (scallions), trimmed and chopped

2 tbsp light mayonnaise

2 wholemeal pitta breads

a large handful of salad leaves

½ red or yellow (bell) pepper, deseeded and chopped

¼ small cucumber, cubed

1 juicy tomato, cut into chunks

4 black olives, stoned (pitted) and sliced

salt and freshly ground black pepper

1. Cook the green beans in a saucepan of boiling water for 3–4 minutes until just tender but still firm. Drain and rinse under cold running water.

2. Meanwhile, cook the eggs in a saucepan of boiling water for 8 minutes. Place in a bowl of cold water and set aside until they are cold, then peel and quarter.

3. Mash the tuna with a fork in a bowl and mix with the spring onions (scallions) and mayonnaise. Season to taste with black pepper.

4. Make a slit down the long side of each pitta bread and gently open it up to make a 'pocket' for the filling. Fill with the tuna mayo, salad leaves, red or yellow (bell) pepper, cucumber, tomato, olives and quartered eggs, then season to taste. Enjoy!

◦ VARIATION:

· Try this as a salad without the pitta. It's great with some crusty bread or you can leave the tuna chunks whole and mix in some cooked baby new potatoes or pasta shapes.

Bean, Tuna & Egg Salad

460kcals PER SERVING | ||| SERVES 2 | ⏱ PREP TIME 15 MIN | 🍲 COOKING TIME 7 MIN

Everyone has their own preferred way of boiling eggs, but the correct way to cook them is to boil them until the whites are set but the yolks are still runny, okay? Glad that's settled.

1 x 200g/7oz can tuna in spring
  water, drained
1 x 200g/7oz can red kidney beans,
  rinsed and drained
4 spring onions (scallions), trimmed
  and chopped
1 small bag of salad leaves
200g/7oz fine green beans, trimmed
2 medium free-range eggs
salt and freshly ground black pepper

DRESSING
2 tbsp olive oil
2 tbsp cider or red wine vinegar
1 tbsp honey mustard
a good squeeze of lemon juice

1. Break the tuna into pieces and place in a bowl with the kidney beans, spring onions (scallions) and salad leaves.
2. Make the dressing: mix all the ingredients together in a bowl or shake in a screw-top jar until well combined.
3. Cook the green beans in a saucepan of lightly salted boiling water for 2 minutes until they are just tender but still retain some bite. Drain and refresh under cold running water. Set aside.
4. Bring a separate saucepan of water to the boil and carefully add the eggs. Boil for 5 minutes then remove from the pan with a slotted spoon. Leave to cool for a moment or cool under cold running water, then peel them.
5. Add the green beans to the tuna salad mixture and toss together gently with the dressing. Season to taste with salt and pepper.
6. Divide the salad between two serving plates or bowls. Cut the boiled eggs in half lengthways and serve on top of the salad.

Warm Lentil & Mozzarella Salad with Pesto

405kcals PER SERVING | ⫴ SERVES 2 | ⏱ PREP TIME 10 MIN | 🍲 COOKING TIME 30 MINS

This salad is best served lukewarm or at room temperature rather than cold from the fridge. And please don't use red lentils to make it as they collapse when cooked and don't retain their shape. I learned that the mushy way.

100g (4oz/½ cup) Puy or green lentils
(dry weight)
1 tbsp olive oil
1 onion, chopped
2 carrots, finely diced
2 celery sticks, diced
2 garlic cloves, crushed
150g/5oz baby plum tomatoes,
halved
juice of 1 lemon
a handful of parsley or basil, leaves
chopped
2 tbsp balsamic vinegar
100g/4oz fine green beans, trimmed
60g/2oz mozzarella, sliced
2 tsp fresh green pesto
salt and freshly ground black pepper

1. Put the lentils into a saucepan and cover them with cold water. Bring to the boil, then reduce the heat and simmer gently for about 20 minutes until they are just tender but still retain some bite. Drain and refresh under cold running water.

2. Meanwhile, heat the oil in a large deep frying pan (skillet) set over a low heat. Add the onion, carrots, celery and garlic and cook gently, stirring occasionally, for about 10 minutes until softened.

3. Stir in the tomatoes and cooked lentils and cook for 5 minutes, stirring occasionally. If the lentils start to stick to the pan, add a little water or vegetable stock. Stir in the lemon juice, herbs and balsamic vinegar. Season to taste with salt and pepper, then remove from the heat and set aside to cool.

4. Cook the green beans in a saucepan of boiling water for about 3 minutes until just tender. Drain and refresh under cold running water. Pat dry with kitchen paper (paper towels).

5. Divide the lentil salad between two serving plates. Top with the mozzarella and green beans, and drizzle with pesto.

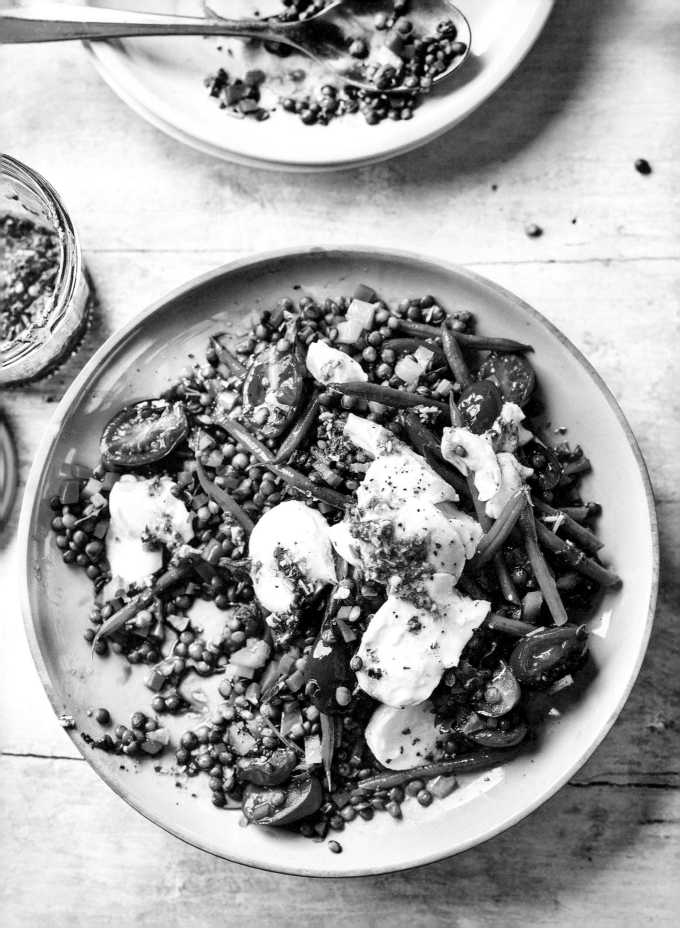

Chickpea & Couscous Salad with Tahini Drizzle

525kcals PER SERVING | ⊪ SERVES 2 | ⏱ PREP TIME 15 MIN | 🍲 COOKING TIME 25-35 MIN

Eat this warm for a light lunch or for tea. Try it cold as a packed lunch, too. Also try varying the roasted vegetables you use – beetroot, courgettes or tomatoes, for example, work just as well.

1 red onion, cut into wedges

1 red or yellow (bell) pepper, deseeded and cut into chunks

1 small aubergine (eggplant) or fennel bulb, sliced

2 tbsp olive oil

100g (4oz/scant 1 cup) giant couscous

150ml (5fl oz/scant ¾ cup) vegetable stock

grated zest and juice of 1 lemon

2 tbsp pine nuts

200g (7oz/¾ cup) canned chickpeas (garbanzo beans), rinsed and drained

a handful of flat-leaf parsley or mint, chopped

salt and freshly ground black pepper

TAHINI DRIZZLE

120g (4½oz/½ cup) natural low-fat yoghurt

2 tsp tahini

1 garlic clove, crushed

1 tsp olive oil

grated zest and juice of ½ lemon

1. Preheat the oven to 180°C/160°C fan/350°F/gas 4.

2. Put the red onion, (bell) pepper and aubergine or fennel in a roasting pan and drizzle with the olive oil. Season lightly with salt and pepper, then roast in the oven for 25–30 minutes until tender.

3. Meanwhile, make the tahini drizzle: put all the ingredients in a bowl and mix together well, seasoning to taste with salt and pepper.

4. Cook the couscous, according to the packet instructions, in the vegetable stock. Fluff it up with a fork and stir in the lemon zest and juice. Season to taste and transfer to a serving bowl.

5. Set a small heavy-based frying pan (skillet) over a medium–high heat, add the pine nuts and toast, tossing them occasionally, for 2 minutes until golden brown. Remove from the pan immediately.

6. Stir the roasted vegetables (and their oil) into the cooked couscous with the chickpeas and herbs. Drizzle with the tahini mixture and sprinkle with the toasted pine nuts. Serve warm or cold.

💡 **TIP:** If you can't find any giant couscous, use the regular sort and just follow the cooking instructions on the packet.

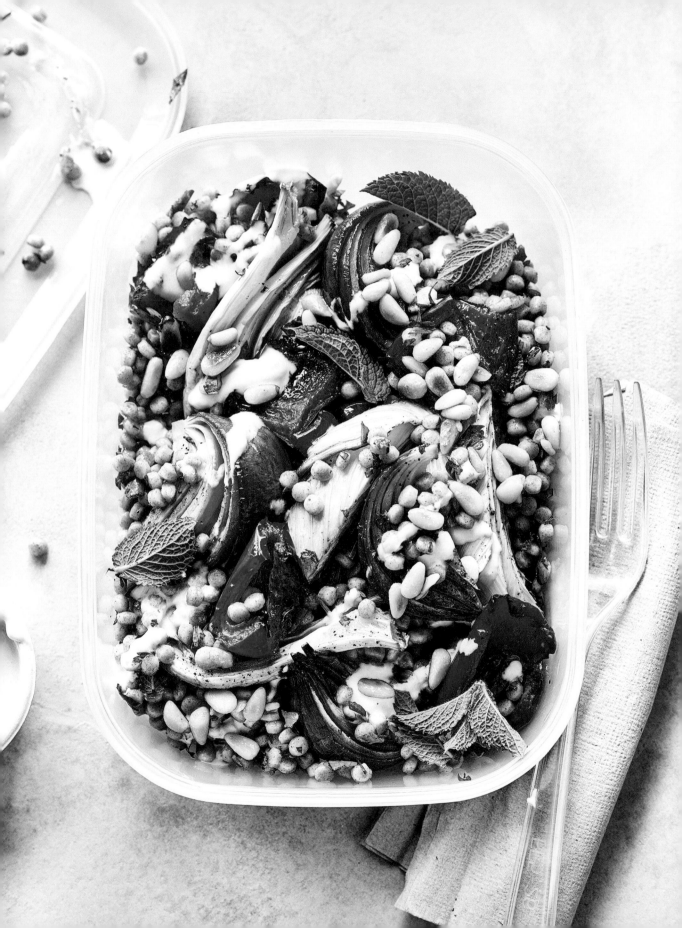

Lamb Kofta Pittas with Tzatziki

360kcals PER SERVING | ▐▊▐ SERVES 2 | ⏱ PREP TIME 15 MIN | 🍲 COOKING TIME 10 MIN

You can use extra-lean minced beef instead of lamb to make the kofta if you prefer, which will save approximately 30kcals per serving. If I'm in a hurry, I cheat and use ready-made supermarket tzatziki. If you do that though, make sure to recalculate the calorie count!

225g (8oz/generous 1 cup) extra-lean minced (ground) lamb (maximum 5% fat)
2 garlic cloves, crushed
½ tsp ground coriander
a pinch of ground cumin
a few sprigs of mint, leaves chopped
grated zest and juice of ½ lemon
salt and freshly ground black pepper

TZATZIKI
125g (4½oz/½ cup) 0% fat Greek yoghurt
¼ cucumber, diced
1 garlic clove, crushed
juice of ½ lemon
a few sprigs of mint, leaves chopped

TO SERVE
2 wholemeal pitta breads
a few crisp salad leaves
1 juicy tomato, sliced
lemon wedges

1. Mix together the lamb, garlic, ground spices, mint, lemon zest and juice and a little seasoning in a bowl. Divide into 6 portions and, using your hands, shape each one into a ball. Preheat the grill (broiler) to high.

2. Thread the balls onto two thin wooden or bamboo skewers, which have been soaked in water to prevent them burning (see Tip on page 104). Place on a metal rack standing in a foil-lined grill (broiler) pan and cook under the preheated grill for about 10 minutes, turning them occasionally, until cooked and appetizingly brown all over.

3. Meanwhile, mix the tzatziki ingredients together in a bowl and season to taste.

4. Warm the pitta breads in a griddle pan or low oven and split each one along the side to open it up and make a 'pocket'. Remove the kofta balls from the skewers and place inside the pittas with some salad leaves and tomato slices. Top with the tzatziki and serve immediately with lemon wedges for squeezing.

💡 **TIP:** If you love hot, spicy food, add 1 teaspoon curry powder to the kofta mix or drizzle the filled pittas with some sweet chilli sauce (1 tablespoon per person will add about 35kcals to each serving).

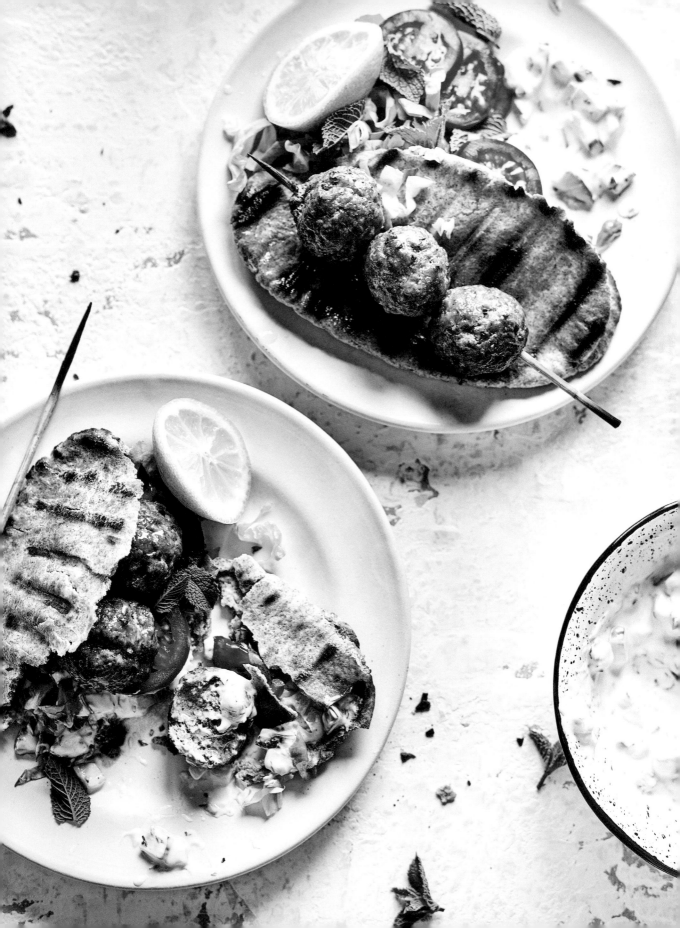

Chicken & Hummus Wraps

490kcals PER SERVING | ||| SERVES 2 | ⏱ PREP TIME 10 MIN | 🍲 COOKING TIME 15 MIN

This is one of those lunches that feels so filling and 'big' that you wonder how it can possibly be healthy, but it absolutely is (plus at least you know what's gone in these rather than the pre-packed supermarket versions). You can make the chicken and red pepper mixture the night before and chill in the fridge overnight, then just add the hummus, carrot and herbs the following day before serving cold or popping into a lunckbox.

1 tbsp olive oil

200g/7oz chicken breast fillets, cut into strips

1 red (bell) pepper, deseeded and cut into strips

2 garlic cloves, crushed

1 small red chilli, deseeded and diced

2 wholemeal tortilla wraps

100g (4oz/½ cup) hummus

1 carrot, grated

juice of ½ lemon

a handful of coriander (cilantro), chopped

salt and freshly ground black pepper

1. Heat the oil in a frying pan (skillet) set over a medium heat. Add the chicken strips and red (bell) pepper and cook, turning occasionally, for 8–10 minutes until the chicken is golden brown and cooked through and the red pepper is tender. Add the garlic and chilli and cook for 1 minute. Remove and keep warm.
2. Meanwhile, heat the wraps in the microwave or warm them in a griddle pan.
3. Spread the hummus over the wraps and top with the grated carrot and chicken and red pepper mixture. Sprinkle with the lemon juice and coriander (cilantro) and season lightly with salt and pepper.
4. Fold the wraps over the filling to enclose it or roll them up and eat immediately while still warm.

💡 VARIATIONS:

· Add some Greek yoghurt, cumin or caraway seeds to the wraps before rolling them up.
· Use as a filling for a sandwich or pitta pocket.

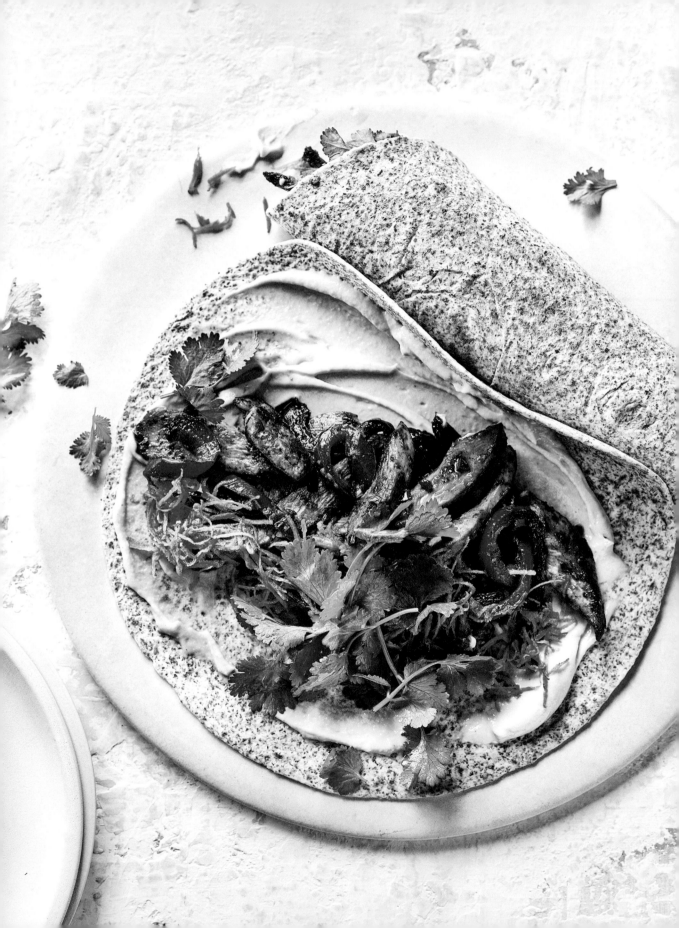

Tandoori Chicken Wraps

420kcals PER SERVING | ||| SERVES 2 | ⏱ PREP TIME 15 MIN | 🍲 COOKING TIME 10-15 MIN

This is one of my favourite meals to make when I've got a friend coming round. Incredibly healthy, yet filling, it looks as good as it tastes. You will need four wooden skewers.

2 tbsp tandoori paste

120g (4½oz/½ cup) 0% fat Greek yoghurt

225g/8oz chicken breast fillets, cut into chunks

2 x 45g/1½oz wholemeal wraps or low-fat chapatis

6 cherry tomatoes, halved

¼ red onion, diced

a few crisp lettuce leaves, shredded

salt and freshly ground black pepper

CUCUMBER RAITA

200g (7oz/scant 1 cup) 0% fat Greek yoghurt

leaves from a handful of mint, chopped

¼ cucumber, diced

1 garlic clove, crushed

3 spring onions (scallions), trimmed and finely chopped

a good pinch of ground cumin

a pinch of ground coriander

1. Mix the tandoori paste and yoghurt together in a bowl. Add the chicken and stir gently until it's well coated. Cover and chill in the fridge for at least 30 minutes.
2. Make the raita: mix all the ingredients together in a bowl, season with salt and pepper, then cover and chill in the fridge. Preheat the grill (broiler) to high.
3. Thread the marinated chicken onto four wooden skewers and place in a foil-lined grill (broiler) pan. Cook under the preheated grill, turning occasionally, for 10–15 minutes until cooked through and golden brown outside. Alternatively, cook on a hot barbecue or in a griddle pan.
4. Warm the wraps or chapatis in a griddle pan or low oven.
5. Slide the chicken off the skewers and place on top of the warm wraps or chapatis with the tomatoes, diced onion and shredded lettuce. Spoon the raita over the top and fold over or roll up. Serve warm.

💡 **TIP:** Soak the wooden skewers in warm water for 30 minutes before using them. This will prevent them burning under the grill.

Chicken & Aubergine Stacks

325kcals PER SERVING | 🍴 SERVES 2 | ⏱ PREP TIME 15 MIN | 🍲 COOKING TIME 6-12 MIN

Aubergine's firm, meaty texture lends itself to griddling or barbecuing.

2 medium aubergines (eggplants),
   topped and tailed

2 tsp olive oil

300g/10oz cooked chicken breast
   fillets, diced

1 small ripe avocado, peeled, stoned
   (pitted) and diced

2 tbsp 0% fat Greek yoghurt

2 tbsp finely chopped parsley

a squeeze of lemon juice

salt and freshly ground black pepper

1. Cut each aubergine (eggplant) into 4 chunky rounds, about 1cm/½in thick. Brush them with the oil and season lightly.

2. Heat a griddle pan over a medium-high heat then add the aubergine slices (cook in batches if necessary). Cook for about 3 minutes on each side until golden brown. Drain on kitchen paper (paper towels).

3. Meanwhile, mix together the chicken, avocado, yoghurt, parsley and lemon juice in a bowl. Season to taste.

4. To assemble the stacks, place a slice of aubergine on a plate then add a layer of chicken. Cover with another aubergine slice and keep layering, finishing with a layer of chicken. You will have 2 stacks, each with 4 aubergine slices. Serve immediately.

Steak with Paprika Avocado Dip

385kcals PER SERVING | 🍴 SERVES 2 | ⏱ PREP TIME 10 MIN | 🍲 COOKING TIME 5-10 MIN

A juicy protein, vitamin, and mineral-rich steak is so quick and easy to cook.

2 x 150g/5oz lean rump, sirloin or
   fillet steaks

olive oil, for brushing

100g/4oz spinach, washed and trimmed

salt and freshly ground black pepper

PAPRIKA AVOCADO DIP

1 small ripe avocado, peeled and
   stoned (pitted)

2 tbsp 0% fat Greek yoghurt

1 tsp sweet paprika

a squeeze of lemon juice

1. Make the paprika avocado dip: use a fork to mash the avocado flesh with the yoghurt and paprika in a bowl. Add the lemon juice, season and set aside.

2. Lightly brush both sides of the steaks with oil and season with salt and pepper.

3. Heat a griddle pan over a high heat, then add the steaks. For rare meat, cook for 1-2 minutes on each side; for medium, 3 minutes on each side; and for well done, 4 minutes on each side. Remove from the griddle and leave to rest for 2-3 minutes.

4. Steam the spinach for 2 minutes until wilted.

5. Serve the warm steaks and spinach with the paprika avocado dip.

Chicken Laksa Bowl

430kcals PER SERVING | ᵧᵧᵧ SERVES 4 | ⏱ PREP TIME 15 MIN | 🍲 COOKING TIME 15-20 MIN

This recipe makes four servings so that's lunch sorted for Monday to Thursday! Plus, there's something immensely satisfying about eating a whole meal in a bowl, right?

1 tbsp vegetable or groundnut (peanut) oil

a bunch of spring onions (scallions), trimmed and sliced

250g/9oz mushrooms, sliced

3 garlic cloves, crushed

2 tsp peeled and finely diced fresh root ginger

1 red chilli, thinly sliced

1 stalk lemongrass, peeled and tender part diced

1 litre (1¾ pints/4¼ cups) hot chicken stock

200ml (7fl oz/generous ¾ cup) canned reduced-fat coconut milk

1 tbsp nam pla (Thai fish sauce)

400g/14oz cooked skinned chicken breasts, sliced

100g (4oz/1 cup) bean sprouts

150g/5oz rice noodles (dry weight)

juice of 1 lime

salt and freshly ground black pepper

a few sprigs of Thai basil or coriander (cilantro), chopped, to serve

1. Heat the oil in a deep frying pan (skillet) or wok set over a medium-high heat, add the spring onions (scallions), mushrooms, garlic, ginger, chilli and lemongrass and stir-fry for 2–3 minutes. Add the hot stock, coconut milk and nam pla. Reduce the heat and simmer for 5 minutes, then add the chicken and simmer gently for 5 more minutes until everything is hot.

2. Meanwhile, cook the rice noodles according to the packet instructions and drain well.

3. Stir the bean sprouts and rice noodles into the laksa and season to taste with salt and pepper. Heat through gently for 2–3 minutes until the chicken is cooked through, then stir in the lime juice.

4. Ladle the laksa into shallow serving bowls and serve sprinkled with chopped basil or coriander (cilantro).

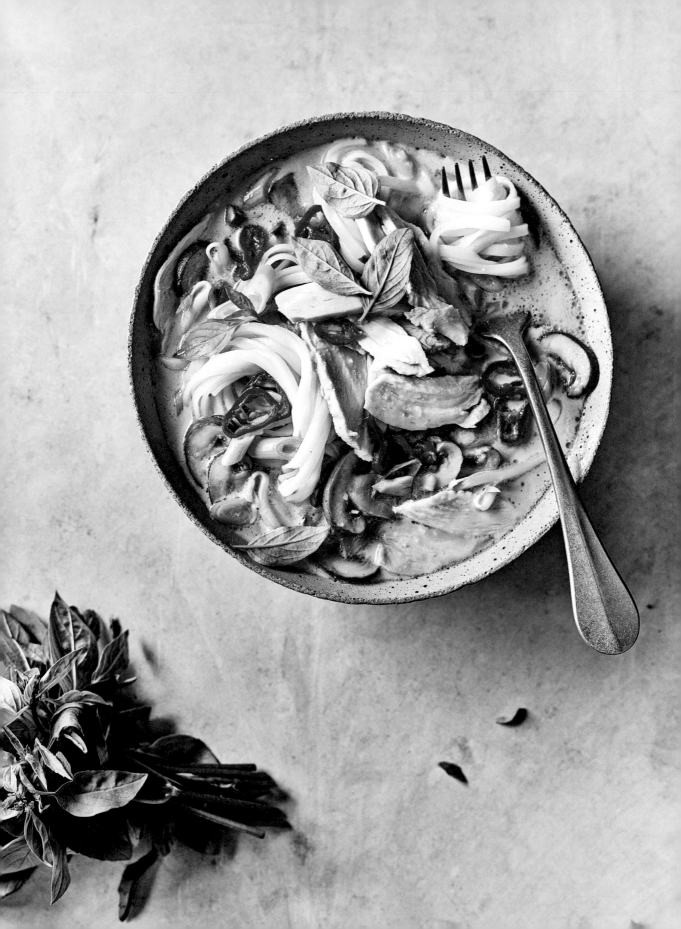

Spiced Sweet Potato Bubble & Squeak

410kcals PER SERVING | ¡¡¡ SERVES 2 | ⏱ PREP TIME 10 MIN | 🍲 COOKING TIME 15-20MIN

This is a great way of using up any leftover cooked root vegetables, like swede, carrots and ordinary potatoes (if you don't have cooked sweet potatoes), as well as greens. Throw them all in for a filling dish that always feels like a treat.

2 tbsp olive oil
1 onion, chopped
2 garlic cloves, crushed
a pinch of dried chilli flakes
1 tsp black mustard seeds
2 tsp ground cumin
1 tsp garam masala or curry powder
300g/10oz cooked sweet potatoes
150g/5oz cooked parsnips
250g/9oz cooked greens, e.g.
    shredded cabbage or kale,
    broccoli, sliced Brussels sprouts
olive oil spray (optional)
2 medium free-range eggs
salt and freshly ground black pepper
hot sauce, for drizzling (optional)

1. Heat the oil in a large non-stick frying pan (skillet) set over a low heat. Add the onion and garlic and cook for 6–8 minutes until softened. Stir in the chilli flakes, mustard seeds and spices and cook for 2 minutes.
2. Meanwhile, mash the sweet potatoes and parsnips roughly, and shred or slice the green vegetables.
3. Add the mashed vegetables to the pan, stirring them into the spicy onion mixture. Season with salt and pepper and press down with a spatula to cover the base and level the top. Cook for 4–5 minutes until crisp and golden brown underneath, then turn the mixture over so the crispy bits are on top. Don't worry if it breaks up – just press it down and flatten it out and cook for a few more minutes until it's heated right through and golden brown underneath.
4. Meanwhile, lightly spray a separate pan with oil and fry the eggs, or poach them to your liking in a pan of gently simmering water.
5. Divide the bubble and squeak between two serving plates and top with the cooked eggs. If wished, drizzle with some hot sauce.

Tuscan Bean & Vegetable Bowl

325kcals PER SERVING | ||| SERVES 4 | ⏱ PREP TIME 15 MIN | 🍲 COOKING TIME 45-55 MIN

Falling halfway between a stew and a soup, this meal-in-a-bowl is a proper comfort dish that will warm you up on cold days and there's hardly any washing up!

1 tbsp olive oil

1 onion, chopped

1 large leek, trimmed, washed and chopped

2 celery sticks, chopped

2 large carrots, diced

2 garlic cloves, crushed

1 litre (1¾ pints/4¼ cups) hot vegetable stock

400g (14oz/2 cups) canned chopped tomatoes

2 medium potatoes, peeled and cubed

2 sprigs of thyme, leaves stripped and chopped

1 sprig of rosemary, leaves stripped and chopped

400g (14oz/2 cups) canned borlotti or cannellini beans, rinsed and drained

180g/6½oz curly kale or Savoy cabbage, shredded

salt and freshly ground black pepper

2 tbsp grated Parmesan cheese, to serve

(V) (GF)

1. Heat the olive oil in a large saucepan set over a low heat, add the onion, leek, celery and carrots and cook, stirring occasionally, for 10 minutes until softened but not browned. Stir in the garlic and cook for 1 minute.

2. Add the stock, tomatoes and potatoes and bring to the boil. Reduce the heat and add the herbs. Simmer gently for 30–40 minutes until the vegetables are tender.

3. Add the beans and kale or cabbage and cook gently for 5 minutes – do not overcook or the kale will become soggy and lose its lovely, bright green freshness. Season to taste with salt and pepper.

4. Serve in shallow bowls sprinkled with grated Parmesan.

💡 VARIATIONS:

· Sprinkle with grated Cheddar cheese instead of Parmesan.

· Stir 1 teaspoon fresh pesto into each bowl just before serving.

· Add a good handful of macaroni or vermicelli about 10 minutes before the end of cooking.

Easy Sweet Potato Fishcakes

495kcals PER SERVING | SERVES 2 | PREP TIME 15 MIN | COOKING TIME 5 MIN

This is a great recipe for using up leftover sweet potato or ordinary mashed potato if you don't want the faff of baking fresh ones. Sometimes I use flaked cold poached salmon or even chopped smoked salmon trimmings. I like to eat the fishcakes with a fresh salad or steamed green vegetables.

400g/14oz sweet potatoes, scrubbed

1 tbsp sunflower or vegetable oil, plus extra for frying

2 large leeks, trimmed, washed and thinly sliced

200g/7oz canned salmon in spring water, drained and flaked

a handful of parsley or chives, finely chopped

1 tbsp teriyaki or light soy sauce

1 tbsp plain (all-purpose) flour, plus extra for dusting

salt and freshly ground black pepper

TO SERVE

sweet chilli sauce, for drizzling

lemon wedges, for squeezing

1. Preheat the oven to 200°C/180°C fan/400°F/gas 6.
2. Pierce the sweet potatoes a few times with a fork. Place on a baking tray (cookie sheet) and bake for 30–40 minutes or until tender when squeezed. Remove and set aside to cool. Alternatively, cook in the microwave.
3. Meanwhile, heat the oil in a frying pan (skillet) set over a low heat, add the leeks and cook for 6–8 minutes until softened but not browned.
4. When the sweet potatoes are cool enough to handle, cut them open, scoop out the insides and mix gently in a bowl with the cooked leeks, salmon, parsley or chives and teriyaki or soy sauce. Stir in the flour to bind everything together and season with salt and pepper.
5. Divide the mixture into 6 portions and shape each one into a patty with your hands. Dust each patty lightly with flour, cover and chill in the fridge for at least 30 minutes to firm up.
6. Heat a little oil – not too much – in a large frying pan set over a medium heat and cook the fishcakes for 4–5 minutes on each side until golden brown and crisp. Serve them drizzled with chilli sauce and with lemon wedges for squeezing.

-💡- **TIP:** You can make the fishcake patties in advance and freeze them in batches. Defrost thoroughly before cooking.

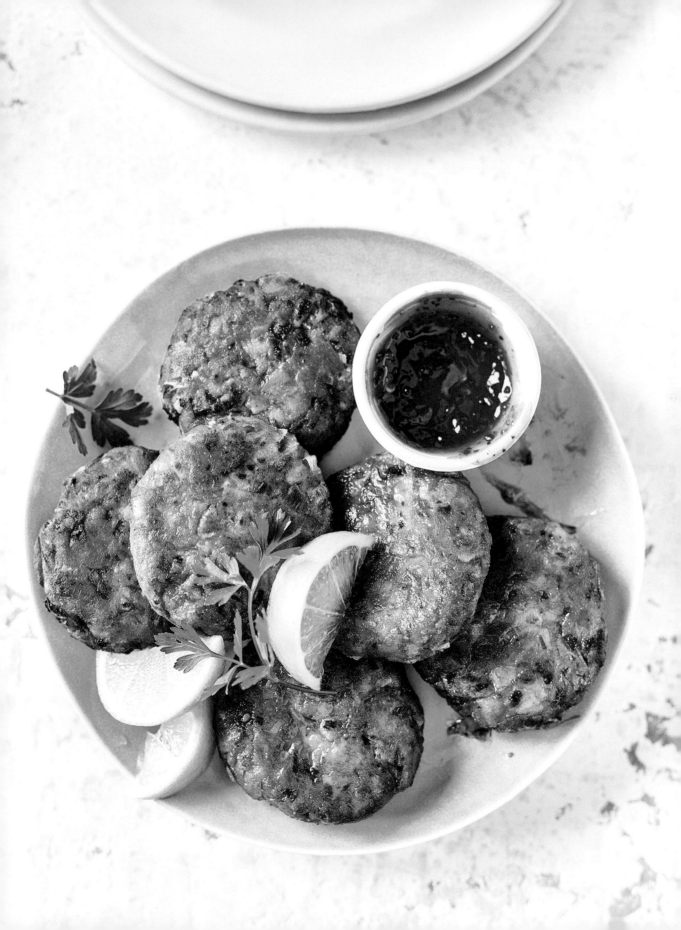

Sweet Potato Jackets with Veggie Chilli

270kcals PER SERVING | ⫴ SERVES 4 | ⏲ PREP TIME 10 MIN | 🍲 COOKING TIME 30-40 MIN

Never baked a sweet potato before? Do it, right now. It'll change your life. You're welcome.

2 medium sweet potatoes, scrubbed
1 tbsp olive oil
1 onion, chopped
2 garlic cloves, crushed
1 red (bell) pepper, deseeded and diced
1 heaped tsp chilli powder
200g (7oz/1 cup) canned chopped
    tomatoes
200g (7oz/1 cup) canned kidney
    beans, rinsed and drained
salt and freshly ground black pepper
50g (2oz/½ cup) Cheddar cheese,
    grated, to serve

1. Preheat the oven to 190°C/170°C fan/375°F/gas 5.
2. Pierce the sweet potatoes a few times with a fork. Bake the sweet potatoes on a baking tray (cookie sheet) for about 45 minutes until tender when you press them gently.
3. Meanwhile, heat the oil in a saucepan set over a low–medium heat. Add the onion, garlic and red (bell) pepper and cook, stirring occasionally, for 6–8 minutes until softened.
4. Stir in the chilli powder and cook for 1 minute, then add the tomatoes and kidney beans. Simmer gently for 10–15 minutes. Season to taste.
5. Split each sweet potato in half. Spoon the chilli over the top and serve sprinkled with the grated cheese.

112

Pea & Roasted Garlic Soup

485kcals PER SERVING | ⫴ SERVES 2 | ⏲ PREP TIME 10 MIN | 🍲 COOKING TIME 45-50 MIN

Cook yourself a vat of homemade soup and snuggle in front of the TV.

1 small head of garlic
2 tbsp olive oil
1 large onion, chopped
1 litre (1¾ pints/4¼ cups) hot
    vegetable stock
500g (1lb 2oz/3½ cups) frozen peas
a handful of mint, roughly chopped
salt and freshly ground black pepper
4 tbsp 0% fat Greek yoghurt, to
    serve
50g (2oz/½ cup) Parmesan cheese,
    grated, to serve

1. Preheat the oven to 200°C/180°C fan/400°F/gas 6.
2. Slice the top off the head of garlic and loosely wrap it, whole and unpeeled, in kitchen foil. Seal the edges of the parcel and roast on a baking tray (cookie sheet) for 30–40 minutes.
3. Meanwhile, heat the oil in a large saucepan set over a low–medium heat. Add the onion and cook for 6–8 minutes, stirring, until softened but not browned. Add the stock and peas and bring to the boil. Reduce the heat and simmer for 10 minutes until the peas are soft. Set aside.
4. Squeeze the garlic cloves out of their skins into the soup. Add the mint and blitz in a blender or food processor until smooth. Reheat and season to taste. Add a swirl of yoghurt and sprinkle with Parmesan.

Spicy Pumpkin & Butterbean Soup

365kcals PER SERVING | ⫸ SERVES 4 | ⏱ PREP TIME 10 MIN | 🍲 COOKING TIME 35 MIN

I make this warming spicy soup in the autumn when there are piles of pumpkins in the super-markets and farmers' markets, but it tastes just as good made with butternut squash or sweet potatoes instead. It also keeps in the freezer for up to three months so make the most of your Tupperware. I like to top it with crushed tortilla chips and some grated cheese but anything goes, so you could just swirl in a spoonful of yoghurt or sprinkle over some chopped herbs.

2 tbsp olive oil

1 large onion, finely chopped

3 garlic cloves, crushed

1 large carrot, thinly sliced

1kg/2¼lb pumpkin, peeled, deseeded and cubed

a pinch of dried chilli flakes

1 tsp smoked paprika

1 tsp ground turmeric

½ tsp ground nutmeg

1.2 litres (2 pints/5 cups) hot vegetable stock

400g (14oz/2 cups) canned butterbeans (lima beans), rinsed and drained

salt and freshly ground black pepper

TO SERVE

50g/2oz tortilla chips, roughly crushed

50g (2oz/½ cup) Cheddar cheese, grated

Ⓥ ⒼⒻ

1. Heat the oil in a large saucepan set over a low heat. Add the onion and garlic and cook for 6–8 minutes until it starts to soften. Add the carrot and pumpkin and cook, stirring occasionally, for 5 minutes. Add the chilli flakes and ground spices and cook for 1 minute.

2. Pour in the hot stock and bring to the boil. Reduce the heat and simmer gently for 15 minutes or until the vegetables are tender. Add half of the butterbeans (lima beans) to the soup.

3. Blitz in batches, in a blender or food processor, until smooth. Alternatively, purée the soup in the pan, off the heat, with an electric hand-held blender.

4. Return the soup to the pan and stir in the rest of the beans. Season to taste with salt and pepper and heat gently.

5. Ladle into bowls and serve sprinkled with the tortilla chips and grated Cheddar.

💡 **VARIATION:**

· Swap the butterbeans for other white canned beans, such as cannellini or haricot (navy) beans.

Soupe au Pistou

400kcals PER SERVING | SERVES 4 | PREP TIME 10 MIN | COOKING TIME 35 MIN

This healthy summer vegetable soup from Provence is packed with more nutritional good stuff than you can shake a stick (of celery) at. I can't get enough of it. You can make it into a more hefty meal-in-a-bowl for dinner by adding some soup pasta or orzo.

2 tbsp fruity green olive oil

1 onion, finely chopped

3 garlic cloves, crushed

4 celery sticks, finely chopped

1 large leek, trimmed, washed and chopped

150g/5oz baby turnips, peeled and diced

300g/10oz baby carrots, diced

300g/10oz new potatoes, diced

1 litre (1¾ pints/4¼ cups) hot vegetable stock

4 tomatoes, roughly chopped

400g (14oz/2 cups) canned haricot (navy) beans, rinsed and drained

2 courgettes (zucchini), diced

100g/4oz fine green beans, trimmed and diced

salt and freshly ground black pepper

4 tbsp green pesto, to serve

1. Heat the oil in a large saucepan set over a low heat. Add the onion, garlic, celery, leek, turnips and carrots and cook, stirring occasionally, for about 10 minutes until they start to soften. Add the potatoes and cook for 5 minutes.

2. Pour in the hot stock and add the tomatoes and haricot (navy) beans. Simmer gently for 15 minutes before adding the courgettes (zucchini) and green beans. Cook for another 5 minutes until all the vegetables are tender. Season to taste with salt and pepper.

3. Ladle into four shallow soup bowls and swirl a big dollop of pesto into each serving.

VARIATIONS:

· Add some shredded spring greens or spinach, shelled fresh peas, broad beans (fava), shredded runner beans or diced asparagus.

· Sprinkle the soup with grated Parmesan.

LIGHT MEALS & LUNCHES

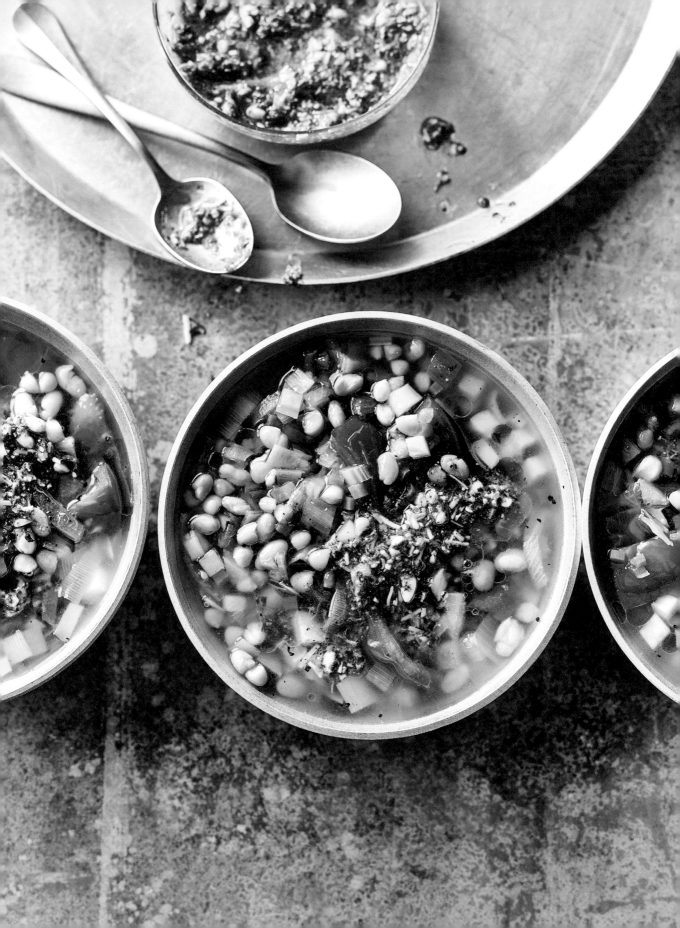

MAIN
MEALS

Veggie Pad Thai with Crunchy Peanuts

630kcals PER SERVING | ⫴ SERVES 2 | ⏲ PREP TIME 10 MIN | 🍲 COOKING TIME 6-8 MIN

This super-speedy dinner is perfect to make after a tough day at work. Simply chuck everything into a wok, stir-fry it and, ta-da! A proper healthy meal within 15–20 minutes.

125g/4½oz flat rice noodles (dry weight)

1 tbsp groundnut (peanut) or vegetable oil

4 garlic cloves, crushed

6 spring onions (scallions), trimmed and sliced

1 red chilli, diced

100g/4oz firm tofu, cubed

2 medium free-range eggs, lightly beaten

grated zest and juice of 1 lime

2 tbsp nam pla (Thai fish sauce)

1 tbsp soy sauce

2 tbsp brown sugar

150g (5oz/1½ cups) bean sprouts

25g (1oz/scant ¼ cup) unsalted roasted peanuts

a handful of coriander (cilantro), chopped

1. Prepare the rice noodles according to the packet instructions.
2. Heat the oil in a wok or deep frying pan (skillet) set over a high heat. Add the garlic, spring onions (scallions) and chilli and stir-fry briskly for 1 minute. Add the tofu and stir-fry for 2–3 minutes until golden and crisp.
3. Add the cooked rice noodles and stir-fry for 1–2 minutes, then push everything to the side and add the beaten egg. Cook for 1 minute, stirring until it scrambles. Stir the egg into the noodle mixture with the lime zest and juice, nam pla, soy sauce, brown sugar, bean sprouts and peanuts. Stir-fry for 1–2 minutes.
4. Sprinkle with coriander (cilantro), divide between two shallow serving bowls and eat immediately.

💡 TIP: If you're not vegetarian, you can use raw peeled prawns (shrimp) instead of tofu – make sure they're completely pink and cooked all the way through.

MAIN MEALS

Griddled Piri Piri Prawn Salad

520kcals PER SERVING | ŶŶŶ SERVES 2 | ⏱ PREP TIME 45 MIN | 🍲 COOKING TIME 35–40 MIN

This salad, with a spicy piri piri marinade, is ridiculously easy to make yet looks impressive and tastes great served with herby, lemony potato wedges.

250g/9oz large peeled raw prawns (jumbo shrimp), tails left on

2 garlic cloves, crushed

1 tbsp hot chilli sauce

1 tsp smoked paprika

grated zest and juice of ½ lemon

a handful of crisp salad leaves

175g/6oz cherry tomatoes, halved

4 spring onions (scallions), trimmed and chopped

1 small ripe avocado, peeled, stoned (pitted) and cubed

2 tbsp vinaigrette dressing

LEMON AND HERB POTATOES

400g/14oz new potatoes, halved or quartered

olive oil spray

grated zest and juice of 1 lemon

leaves from a few sprigs of rosemary, oregano or thyme

salt and freshly ground black pepper

1. Preheat the oven to 200°C/180°C fan/400°F/gas 6.

2. Put the prawns (shrimp) in a bowl. Mix together the garlic, chilli sauce, paprika, lemon zest and juice and pour it over the prawns. Stir well, cover and chill in the fridge for at least 30 minutes.

3. Spray the potatoes lightly with oil and toss in a bowl with the lemon zest and juice, herbs and some salt and pepper. Place on a large sheet of kitchen foil, folding the foil loosely over the top and twisting the edges to seal it into a loose parcel. Place on a baking tray (cookie sheet) and cook in the oven for 30–35 minutes until tender. Open the foil parcel halfway through to turn the potatoes and to brown them.

4. When the potatoes are ready, cook the marinated prawns in a hot oiled griddle pan over a medium–high heat for 4–5 minutes, turning halfway, until pink and cooked right through.

5. Toss the salad leaves, tomatoes, spring onions (scallions) and avocado in the dressing and divide between two serving plates. Top with the griddled prawns and serve with the potato wedges.

💡 TIPS:

· Why not fire up the barbecue and cook the potatoes in their foil parcel as well as the prawns over the hot coals? The potatoes will take about 30 minutes to cook.

· I keep a spray diffuser filled with olive oil on the kitchen worktop for frying and roasting chicken, fish and vegetables. It gives ingredients a much more even-coating of oil than dolloping from a bottle, and is healthier too (as you use less).

MAIN MEALS

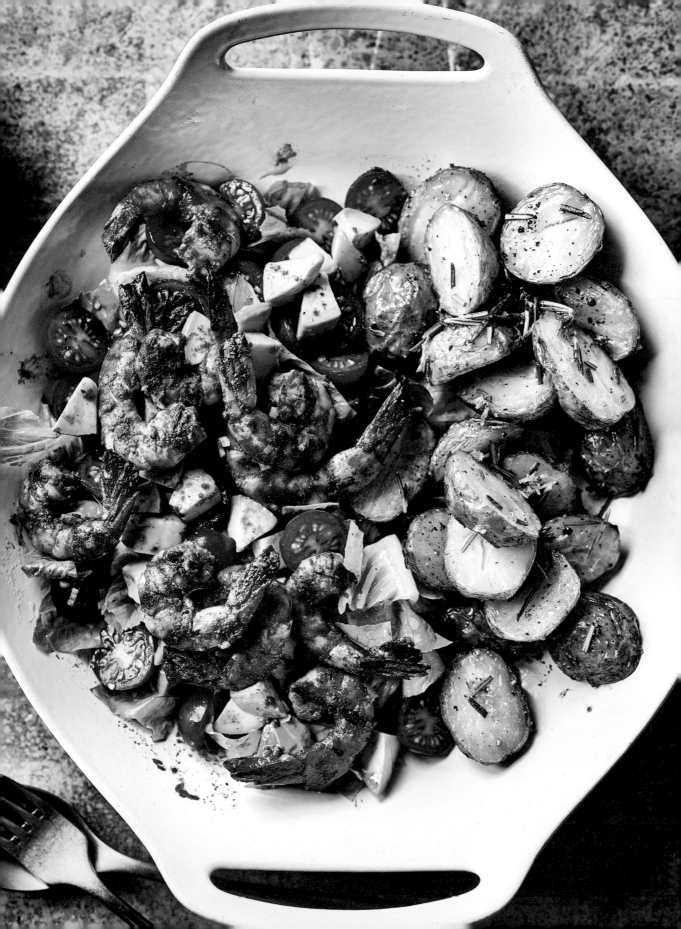

Sesame Chicken with Stir-fried Greens & Noodles

570kcals PER SERVING | ⫙ SERVES 2 | ⏱ PREP TIME 15 MIN | COOKING TIME 10 MIN

This recipe works just as well with whole skinned chicken thighs instead of breasts, but just bear in mind they'll take longer to cook.

85g/3oz rice noodles (dry weight)

1 tbsp dark soy sauce

1 tbsp hoisin sauce

2 tsp runny honey

1 tbsp sesame oil

a pinch of salt

2 x 125g/4½oz chicken breast fillets, thickly sliced

50g (2oz/generous ¼ cup) white sesame seeds

2.5cm/1in piece of fresh root ginger, peeled and shredded

2 garlic cloves, thinly sliced

1 red chilli, shredded

1 tsp cumin seeds

a small bunch of spring onions (scallions), trimmed and sliced diagonally

250g/9oz spring greens, spinach or pak choi (bok choy), shredded

2 tsp light soy sauce or nam pla (Thai fish sauce)

1. Cook the rice noodles according to the packet instructions.

2. Meanwhile, in a large bowl, mix together the dark soy and hoisin sauces, honey, 1 teaspoon of the sesame oil and the salt. Add the chicken and coat it all over with the mixture, then dip the chicken slices into the sesame seeds in a shallow bowl until thoroughly coated.

3. Heat most of the remaining sesame oil in a wok or deep frying pan (skillet) set over a medium heat. When it's hot, add the sesame coated chicken and cook for about 3 minutes on each side until richly browned and slightly sticky and the chicken is cooked right through. Remove from the heat and keep warm.

4. Heat the remaining oil in a clean wok or pan over a medium–high heat, add the ginger, garlic, chilli and cumin seeds and stir-fry for 2 minutes or until the seeds start to crackle. Add the spring onions (scallions), greens and soy sauce or nam pla and stir-fry briskly for 2 minutes.

5. Divide the rice noodles between two serving plates and add the stir-fried spring greens. Place the sesame chicken on top.

MAIN MEALS

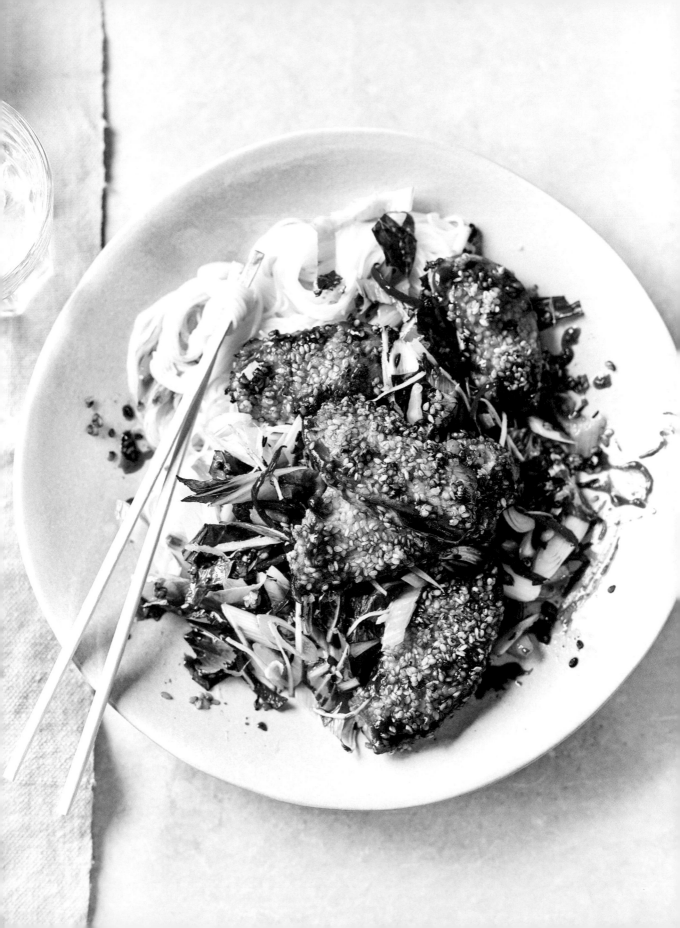

Pan-fried Turkey with Red Cabbage Slaw

595kcals PER SERVING | ⑪ SERVES 2 | ⏲ PREP TIME 25 MIN | 🍲 COOKING TIME 45 MIN

If you've ever had one foot in the 'turkey is boring' camp, this recipe will teach you the error of your ways. It's lean, healthy, protein-rich and really tasty when paired with the red cabbage slaw and sweet potatoes.

2 medium sweet potatoes, scrubbed
100g (4oz/1½ cups) fresh white
　breadcrumbs
1 tbsp grated Parmesan cheese
a few sprigs of sage, leaves finely
　chopped
grated zest of 1 lemon
2 x 100g/4oz turkey breast steaks
1 tsp plain (all-purpose) flour
1 small free-range egg, beaten
1 tbsp olive oil
salt and freshly ground black pepper

RED CABBAGE SLAW
¼ small red cabbage, shredded
¼ red onion, grated
½ small fennel bulb, thinly sliced or
　shredded
2 oranges, 1 peeled, segmented and
　chopped, 1 juiced
1 tbsp olive oil
1 tbsp balsamic vinegar

1. Preheat the oven to 190°C/170°C fan/375°F/gas 5.

2. Pierce the sweet potatoes a few times with a fork. Put them on a baking tray (cookie sheet) and bake in the oven for about 45 minutes or until tender when you press them gently. Remove and set aside to cool. Alternatively, cook in the microwave.

3. Meanwhile, make the red cabbage slaw: put the vegetables and chopped orange in a bowl. Mix together the oil, orange juice and balsamic vinegar and gently toss everything together. Season with salt and pepper to taste.

4. Mix the breadcrumbs, Parmesan, sage and lemon zest in a wide, shallow bowl, then season lightly with salt and pepper.

5. Put the turkey between 2 sheets of cling film (plastic wrap) and bash with a rolling pin or meat tenderiser until flattened out to about 5mm (¼in) thick. Dust the turkey with the flour on both sides, then dip first into the beaten egg and then into the breadcrumb mixture until well coated all over.

6. Heat the olive oil in a large frying pan (skillet) set over a medium heat. Add the breaded turkey and cook for about 4 minutes on each side until crisp, golden and cooked through.

7. Serve the turkey with the red cabbage slaw and the baked sweet potatoes.

💡 VARIATION:
· Swap the turkey for chicken breasts, flattening them in the same way.

MAIN MEALS

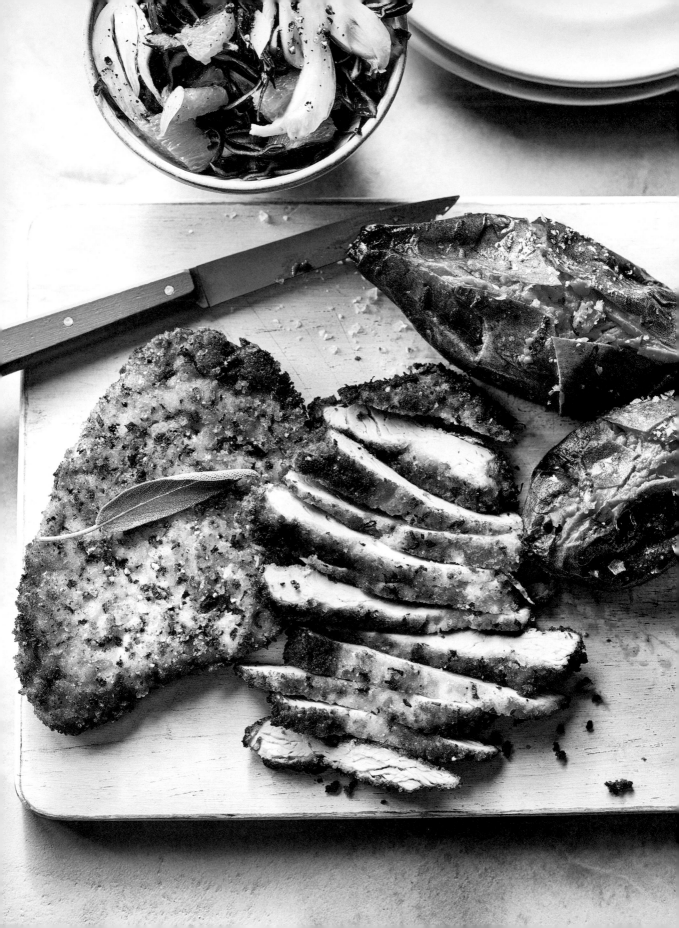

Spicy Chicken Burgers in Sweet Potato Sliders

620kcals PER SERVING | ⬛ SERVES 2 | ⏱ PREP TIME 15 MIN | ⬛ COOKING TIME 30 MIN

A breadless burger can be a bit sad, so whack the patty between two sweet potato slices instead and you've got yourself some healthy buns!

1 large sweet potato, peeled

1 tbsp olive oil, plus extra for
 brushing

225g (8oz/1 cup) minced (ground)
 chicken

½ onion, grated

2 garlic cloves, crushed

2 tsp tomato purée

a little harissa paste (see Tip)

grated zest of 1 lemon

a few sprigs of coriander (cilantro),
 chopped

salt and freshly ground black pepper

FLAGEOLET BEAN SALAD

3 garlic cloves, smashed

a small handful of flat-leaf parsley,
 finely chopped

a small handful of basil, finely
 chopped

2 tbsp olive oil

juice of 1 lemon

400g/14oz canned flageolet beans,
 rinsed and drained

1. Preheat the oven to 200°C/180°C fan/400°F/gas 6.

2. Cut the sweet potato into four thick rounds. Place them on a baking tray (cookie sheet) and drizzle with the oil. Season lightly with salt and pepper, then bake for about 20 minutes until tender but not soft and mushy. The slices must hold their shape.

3. Meanwhile, mix the chicken, onion, garlic, tomato purée, harissa, lemon zest, coriander (cilantro) and some salt and pepper together in a bowl. Divide into two portions and shape each one into a patty. Cover and chill in the fridge for 15 minutes to firm them up.

4. Make the flageolet bean salad: mix together the garlic, herbs, oil and lemon juice in a bowl until you have a green sludgy paste. Warm the beans in their can liquid in a pan, drain, rinse and toss gently in the dressing. Set aside.

5. Set a griddle pan over a medium heat, lightly brush the burgers with oil and cook them in the pan for 5–6 minutes on each side until golden brown and cooked right through. Alternatively, cook on a barbecue or under a hot grill (broiler).

6. Serve the burgers sandwiched between the baked sweet potato slices with the flageolet bean salad.

💡 TIP: Harissa paste is very fiery, so be circumspect and don't use too much. You can always serve some on the side with the cooked burgers.

Lebanese Garlic & Lemon Chicken

595kcals PER SERVING | ᵞᵞᵞ SERVES 2 | ⏱ PREP TIME 20 MIN | 🍲 COOKING TIME 45 MIN

The second best thing about this one-pot dish (the first being how good it tastes, of course),
is there's very little to wash up...

400g/14oz baby new potatoes,
   halved
250g/9oz chicken breast fillets, cut
   into chunks
juice of 2 large lemons
4 unpeeled garlic cloves
½ lemon, cut into slices or wedges
olive oil spray
a good pinch of paprika
a handful of flat-leaf parsley,
   chopped
salt and freshly ground black pepper
harissa, to serve

LEBANESE SALAD
4 ripe tomatoes, chopped
4 radishes, sliced
2 spring onions (scallions), trimmed
   and chopped
¼ cucumber, diced
1 cos (romaine) lettuce, thickly sliced
a handful each of mint and coriander
   (cilantro), chopped
2 tbsp fruity olive oil
1 tbsp pomegranate molasses
juice of ½ lemon
a few drops of balsamic vinegar

GF

1. Preheat the oven to 190°C/170°C fan/375°F/gas 5.
2. Put the potatoes and chicken into a shallow ovenproof dish or roasting pan. Sprinkle with the lemon juice and season with salt and pepper. Tuck in the unpeeled garlic cloves and lemon slices or wedges. Spray lightly with olive oil and stir gently until everything is coated. Dust with the paprika and cover the dish with kitchen foil.
3. Cook in the oven for 30 minutes, then remove the foil and cook for 15 minutes until the potatoes are tender and the chicken is cooked right through and golden brown. Slip the garlic cloves out of their skins and scatter the soft garlic and parsley over the top.
4. Meanwhile, make the salad: mix together the tomatoes, radishes, spring onions (scallions), cucumber, lettuce and herbs in a bowl. Combine the oil, pomegranate molasses, lemon juice and vinegar, pour the mixture over the salad and toss the salad gently in the dressing.
5. Serve the chicken and potatoes with the Lebanese salad and some harissa on the side.

MAIN MEALS

Spicy Salsa Chilli

605kcals PER SERVING | SERVES 2 | PREP TIME 10 MIN | COOKING TIME 45 MIN

Vegetarians can get rid of the mince here and double the amount of kidney beans. Everyone should try this with sliced avocado or homemade guacamole!

2 tsp olive oil

1 onion, finely chopped

1 red (bell) pepper, deseeded and chopped

2 garlic cloves, crushed

200g (7oz/1 cup) extra-lean minced (ground) beef (maximum 5% fat)

2 tsp chilli powder

1 tsp ground cumin

1 tsp sweet paprika

400g (14oz/2 cups) canned chopped tomatoes

240ml (8fl oz/1 cup) beef stock

200g (7oz/generous 1 cup) canned kidney beans, rinsed and drained

100g (4oz/scant ½ cup) canned sweetcorn in water, drained

100g (4oz/½ cup) hot salsa

80g (3oz/generous ⅓ cup) basmati rice (dry weight)

2 tbsp grated Cheddar cheese

salt and freshly ground black pepper

2 tbsp 0% fat Greek yoghurt, to serve

1. Heat the oil in a large saucepan set over a low–medium heat. Add the onion, red (bell) pepper and garlic and cook, stirring occasionally, for 6–8 minutes until softened.

2. Stir in the mince and ground spices and cook, stirring occasionally, for 4–5 minutes until browned all over. Add the tomatoes and stock and bring to the boil.

3. Reduce the heat to a simmer and stir in the kidney beans and sweetcorn. Cook gently for 25–30 minutes or until the beef is cooked, the vegetables are tender and the liquid has reduced and thickened. Stir in the salsa (or spoon it into a bowl to serve separately) and season to taste with salt and pepper.

4. While the chilli is cooking, cook the rice according to the packet instructions.

5. Divide the rice and chilli between two shallow serving bowls and sprinkle with the grated cheese. Add a dollop of Greek yoghurt to each serving and enjoy.

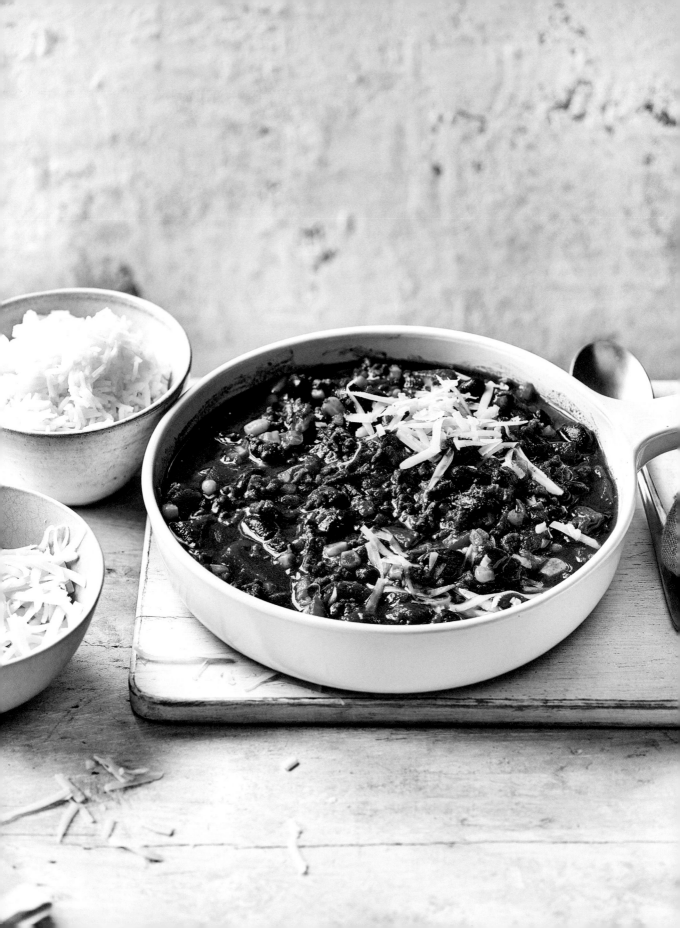

Super Healthy Veggie Burgers

590kcals PER SERVING | ⫴ SERVES 4 | ⏱ PREP TIME 45 MIN | 🍲 COOKING TIME 20 MIN

This recipe is for four veggie burgers because I like to prepare them in advance and then chill them in the fridge overnight, or even freeze them for a later date, before cooking.

500g/1lb 2oz sweet potatoes, peeled and cubed

175g/6oz kale or spring greens, shredded

2 tbsp olive oil

1 small onion, finely chopped

2 garlic cloves, crushed

a small bunch of chives, snipped

50g (2oz/scant ½ cup) roughly chopped roasted hazelnuts or almonds

2 tbsp plain (all-purpose) flour

2 tsp wholegrain mustard

75g/3oz mixed seeds, e.g. pumpkin, sunflower, sesame

salt and freshly ground black pepper

TO SERVE

4 wholemeal rolls or burger buns

sliced tomato and lettuce

tomato ketchup or chilli sauce, for drizzling

1. Cook the sweet potatoes in a saucepan of boiling salted water for about 15 minutes until tender. Drain well and set aside to cool before roughly crushing with a potato masher. Don't worry if it's a bit lumpy.

2. Meanwhile, cook the kale or spring greens in a saucepan of lightly salted boiling water for 4–5 minutes. Drain and roughly chop.

3. Heat 1 tablespoon of the olive oil in a small frying pan (skillet) set over a medium heat, add the onion and garlic and cook for 6–8 minutes, stirring occasionally, until softened. Stir in the chives.

4. Combine the onion mixture in a bowl with the mashed sweet potatoes, cooked greens and nuts. Stir in the flour and mustard and season to taste with salt and pepper. Divide into four portions and use your hands to shape each one into a burger. Roll each burger in the mixed seeds, pressing lightly to coat them all over. Cover and chill in the fridge for at least 30 minutes to firm up.

5. Heat the remaining oil in a non-stick frying pan set over a medium heat. Cook the burgers for 3–4 minutes on each side until crisp and golden brown. Remove and drain on kitchen paper (paper towels).

6. Split and lightly toast the rolls or burger buns. Serve the burgers in the buns with some tomato and lettuce, drizzled with tomato ketchup or chilli sauce.

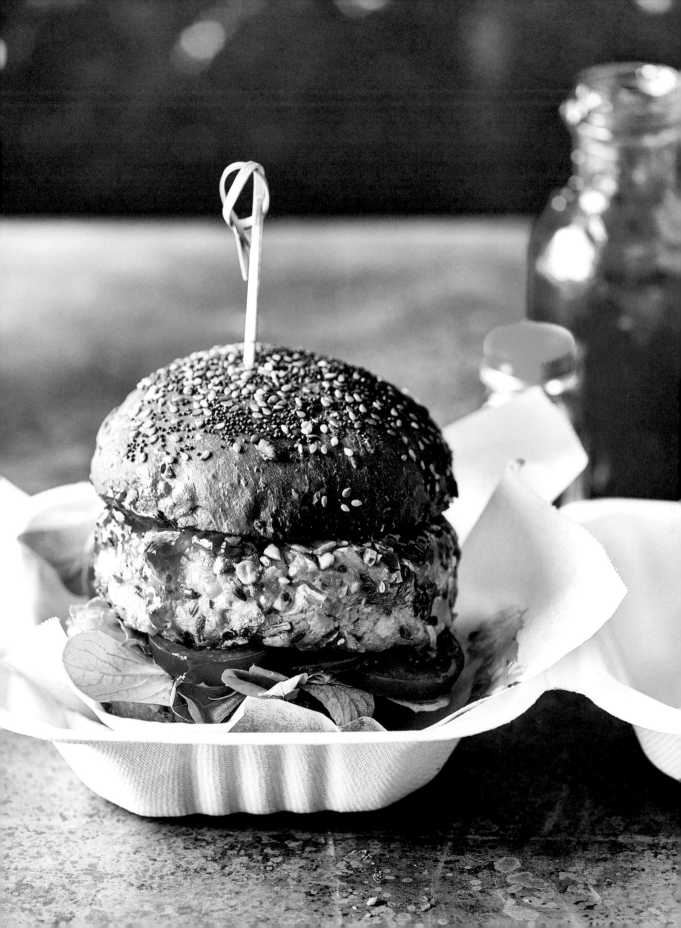

Indian-style Mackerel with Garlicky Green Rice

550kcals PER SERVING | ⫴ SERVES 2 | ⏱ PREP TIME 15 MIN | COOKING TIME 25 MIN

Mackerel is a great source of protein and healthy omega-3 fats, which help protect your heart and boost your brain power! Don't be put off by what seems like a long list of ingredients in this recipe – it really is simple to make.

juice of ½ lime
1 tbsp curry paste
4 tbsp 0% fat Greek yoghurt
2 x 100g/4oz mackerel fillets (with skin)
sunflower oil spray
salt and freshly ground black pepper

SPICY CARROT MASH
400g/14oz carrots, sliced
½ tsp ground cumin
½ tsp ground turmeric
a handful of coriander (cilantro), chopped

GARLICKY GREEN RICE
100g (4oz/scant ½ cup) basmati or brown rice (dry weight)
sunflower oil spray
2 garlic cloves, crushed
1 red chilli, deseeded and shredded
100g/4oz spring greens, green cabbage or kale, shredded

1. Mix together the lime juice, curry paste and yoghurt in a bowl. Slash the skin of the mackerel fillets 2 or 3 times and coat them in the mixture. Cover and chill in the fridge for 30 minutes.
2. Cook the rice according to the packet instructions.
3. Meanwhile, make the spicy carrot mash: cook the carrots in a saucepan of lightly salted boiling water for 10–15 minutes until tender. Drain well, mash with a fork and stir in the ground spices and coriander. Preheat the grill (broiler) to high.
4. Make the garlicky green rice: lightly spray a wok or large frying pan (skillet) with oil and set over a medium–high heat. Add the garlic, chilli and greens and stir-fry for 2–3 minutes, then stir in the cooked rice. Cook briskly, tossing and stirring for a further 1–2 minutes.
5. Remove the mackerel from the marinade and cook in a foil-lined grill (broiler) pan under the preheated grill for 2–3 minutes on each side until cooked and the skin is crisp, brushing it during grilling with the leftover spiced yoghurt mixture.
6. Serve the fish with the spicy carrot mash and garlicky green rice.

MAIN MEALS

Creamy Asparagus & Spinach Pasta

600kcals PER SERVING | ۱۱۱ SERVES 2 | ⏱ PREP TIME 5 MIN | 🍲 COOKING TIME 10 MIN

This quick and easy pasta dish makes a little asparagus go a long way.

200g/7oz tagliatelle or fettuccine
175g/6oz asparagus spears, trimmed
   and cut into 2cm/1in lengths
100g (4oz/scant ½ cup) half-fat
   crème fraîche
grated zest and juice of ½ lemon
100g/4oz baby spinach leaves
1 tbsp poppy seeds
salt and freshly ground black pepper
2 tbsp toasted pine nuts, to serve
2 tbsp grated Parmesan cheese,
   to serve

1. Cook the pasta according to the packet instructions.
2. Steam the asparagus for about 4 minutes until just tender but still firm.
3. Drain the pasta, reserving 2 tablespoons of the cooking water. Return to the warm pan and stir in the crème fraîche and lemon zest. Add the spinach, asparagus and poppy seeds plus the reserved pasta cooking liquid and the lemon juice. Lightly toss everything together and season to taste with salt and pepper. Leave for 1–2 minutes to allow the spinach to wilt into the pasta.
4. Divide between two shallow bowls and serve sprinkled with the pine nuts and Parmesan.

(V)

Flash in the Pan Salmon with Puy Lentils

580kcals PER SERVING | ۱۱۱ SERVES 2 | ⏱ PREP TIME 5 MIN | 🍲 COOKING TIME 20 MIN

One of those dishes that looks really impressive, but takes no time at all to whip up.

150g (5oz/¾ cup) puy lentils (dry
   weight), rinsed in cold water
300ml (½ pint/1¼ cups) stock
1 tbsp olive oil
6 spring onions (scallions), thickly sliced
2 garlic cloves, crushed
2 x 100g/4oz salmon fillets (with skin)
100g (4oz/1½ cups) sunblush
   tomatoes in oil, drained
100g/4oz baby spinach leaves
a few sprigs of parsley, chopped
1–2 tbsp balsamic vinegar
salt and freshly ground black pepper

1. Put the lentils in a saucepan with the stock and set over a high heat. Bring to the boil, then reduce the heat and simmer gently for about 15 minutes.
2. Meanwhile, heat the oil in a non-stick frying pan (skillet) set over a medium heat, add the spring onions (scallions) and garlic and cook for 3 minutes until tender. Remove from the pan and keep warm.
3. Add the salmon to the pan, skin side down, and cook for 5 minutes or until the skin is crisp and golden. Turn it over and cook the other side for 6–8 minutes until cooked through. Remove from the heat.
4. Drain the lentils and return to the pan. Stir in the garlicky spring onions mix, sunblush tomatoes and spinach, folding them through gently, and cook over a low heat for 1 minute. Stir in the parsley and balsamic vinegar and season to taste with salt and pepper. Divide the lentils between two serving plates and place the salmon fillets on top.

Halloumi Kebabs with Smashed Chickpeas

595kcals PER SERVING | ¶¶¶ SERVES 2 | ⏱ PREP TIME 15 MIN | COOKING TIME 12–15 MIN

The great thing about halloumi is that it stays firm when it's cooked, making it perfect for grills and barbecues. I love to thread it onto kebabs with plenty of vegetables.

2 red or yellow (bell) peppers, deseeded and cut into chunks

1 large courgette (zucchini), cut into chunks

4 cherry tomatoes

125g/4½oz halloumi, cubed

olive oil spray

1 tsp sesame seeds

2 tbsp fresh green pesto

salt and freshly ground black pepper

SMASHED CHICKPEAS

400g (14oz/1½ cups) canned chickpeas (garbanzo beans), rinsed and drained

210ml (7fl oz/scant 1 cup) hot vegetable stock

a pinch of ground turmeric

a handful of parsley, mint or coriander (cilantro), chopped

grated zest and juice of ½ lemon

1. Thread the vegetables, tomatoes and halloumi onto six small or four large skewers (if using wooden ones, soak them in water first to prevent them burning – see Tip on page 104). Spray lightly with olive oil and season with salt and pepper. Preheat the grill (broiler) or prepare a barbecue.

2. Cook the kebabs under the preheated grill or on the barbecue for 10–15 minutes, turning them occasionally, until the vegetables are tender and slightly charred around the edges and the halloumi is golden brown.

3. Meanwhile, put the chickpeas (garbanzo beans), hot stock and turmeric in a pan and cook over a low–medium heat for 5 minutes. Drain in a colander, then blitz in a food processor or blender until coarse and grainy. Alternatively, mash roughly with a potato masher. Add the herbs, lemon zest and juice and season to taste with salt and pepper.

4. Sprinkle the kebabs with the sesame seeds. Drizzle with the pesto and serve immediately with the smashed chickpeas.

MAIN MEALS

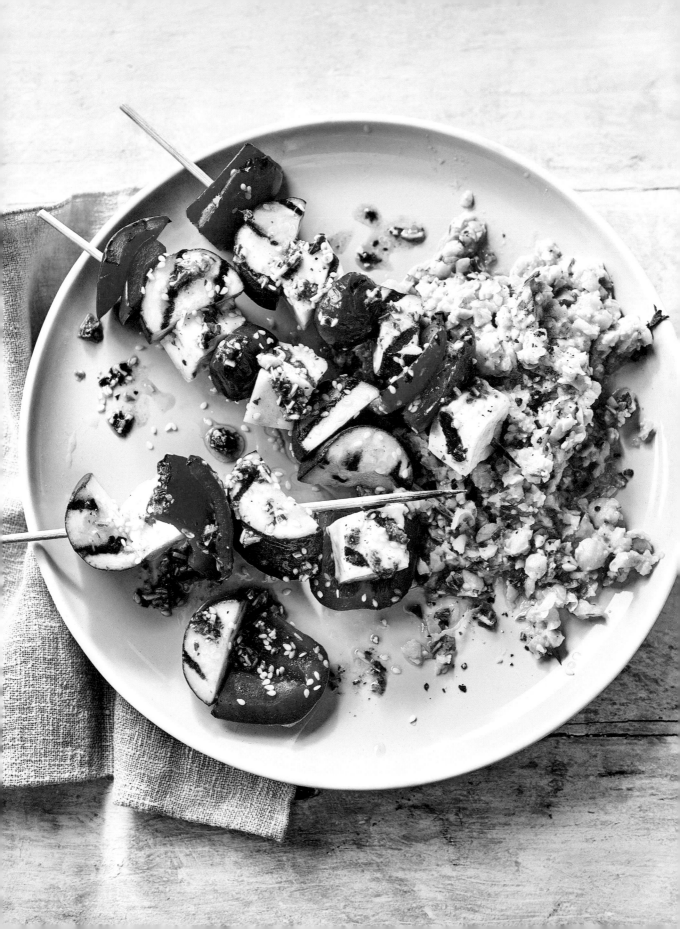

Stir-fried Crispy Tofu & Vegetables

535 kcals PER SERVING | ⟨⟨⟨ SERVES 2 | ⏱ PREP TIME 10 MIN | 🍲 COOKING TIME 10-12 MIN

Tofu (or soya bean curd) is so healthy – packed with protein and minerals, it is especially high in iron and calcium, yet very low in fat. It's also incredibly filling and much cheaper than meat. Win–win. You'll need to use firm tofu for stir-fries so it keeps its shape. If you can't get hold of any pak choi, use broccoli florets instead. I like to serve this with a drizzle of sweet chilli sauce.

200g/7oz firm tofu, cubed

2 tsp cornflour (cornstarch)

1 tbsp sesame or vegetable oil

1 tsp peeled and grated fresh
    root ginger

2 garlic cloves, thinly sliced

1 red chilli, diced

4 spring onions (scallions), trimmed
    and sliced

2 red, yellow or green (bell) peppers,
    deseeded and thinly sliced

200g/7oz pak choi (bok choy), cut
    into quarters lengthways

300g/10oz fresh ready-to-cook rice
    noodles

2 tbsp soy sauce

juice of 1 lime

2 tbsp roasted cashews

salt and freshly ground black pepper

1. Dust the tofu with the cornflour (cornstarch) and season lightly with salt and pepper. Heat the oil in a wok or deep frying pan (skillet) set over a medium–high heat, add the tofu and stir-fry for 4–5 minutes until crisp and golden. Remove with a slotted spoon and drain on kitchen paper (paper towels). Keep warm.

2. Reduce the heat to medium, add the ginger, garlic, chilli and spring onions (scallions) to the wok or pan and stir-fry for 1 minute. Add the (bell) peppers and stir-fry for 2–3 minutes, then stir in the pak choi (bok choy) and noodles. Stir-fry for 2–3 minutes until the noodles are hot and the vegetables are tender but still retain some bite. Add the soy sauce and lime juice and toss to coat.

3. Divide between two shallow serving bowls and top with the crispy tofu and cashews. Eat immediately while it's piping hot.

MAIN MEALS

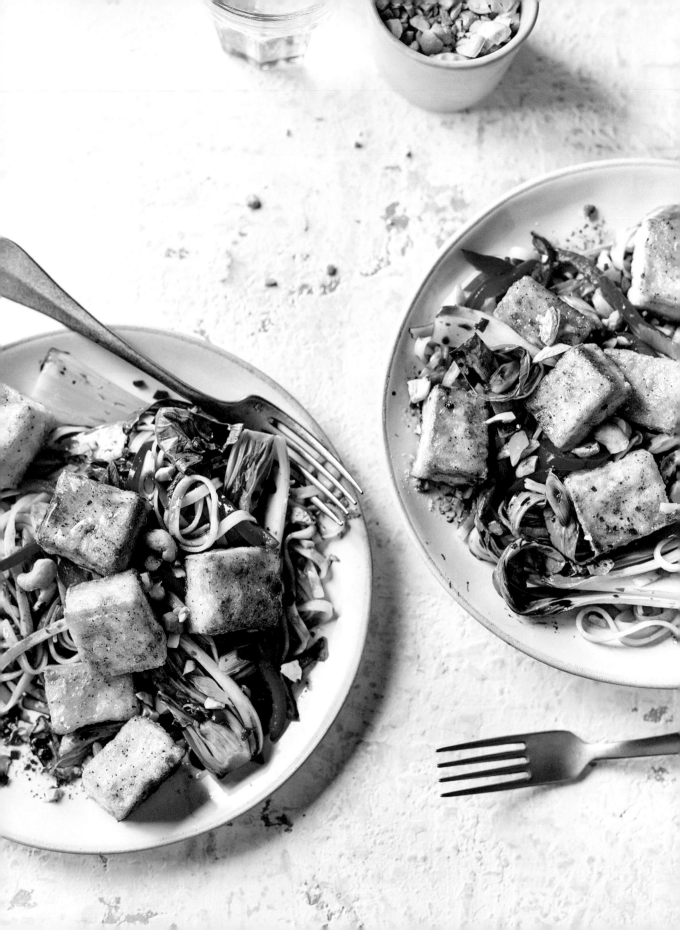

Seedy Roasted Fish Fillets

495kcals PER SERVING | ⑪ SERVES 2 | ⏱ PREP TIME 15 MIN | 🍲 COOKING TIME 25 MIN

You'll need some seeds and spices to make this – I recommend always keeping some to hand in your kitchen cupboard to give a bit of oomph to dishes. They're very healthy and a great way of adding big flavours and extra texture to your food, plus they keep for ages so won't go to waste quickly.

1 tsp coriander seeds

1 tsp black mustard seeds

2 tsp fennel seeds

1 tsp ground turmeric

2 x 175g/6oz thick cod or haddock or cod fillets, skinned

neutral oil, for brushing

salt and freshly ground black pepper

4 tbsp 0% fat Greek yoghurt, to serve

SPICY SPINACH AND SWEET POTATOES

1 tbsp vegetable oil

1cm/½in piece of fresh root ginger, peeled and finely diced or shredded

1 red chilli, deseeded and shredded

1 tsp black mustard seeds

1 tsp cumin seeds

1 tsp ground turmeric

400g/14oz sweet potatoes, peeled and cubed

2 juicy tomatoes, chopped

200g/7oz baby spinach leaves

salt and freshly ground black pepper

1. Preheat the oven to 180°C/160°C fan/350°F/gas 4.

2. Set a frying pan (skillet) over a medium heat and dry-fry the coriander and mustard seeds for 1 minute or until the mustard seeds begin to pop. Stir in the fennel seeds and dry-fry for a further 30 seconds. Remove the seeds from the pan and grind coarsely in a pestle and mortar or electric spice grinder. Add the turmeric and some salt and pepper, and then sprinkle over the fish fillets to coat them.

3. Place the fillets on an oiled baking tray (cookie sheet) and bake in the oven for 15–20 minutes, turning them halfway through, until the spice crust is crisp and golden and the fish is cooked through.

4. While the fish is cooking, make the spicy spinach and potatoes. Heat the oil in a large frying pan set over a medium heat, add the ginger, chilli and seeds and cook for 2 minutes. Stir in the turmeric and sweet potatoes and cook for 5 minutes, stirring occasionally. Add 2–3 tablespoons water and the tomatoes, then cover and simmer gently for about 10 minutes until the potatoes are tender. Stir in the spinach and as soon as it wilts remove the pan from the heat. Season to taste with salt and pepper.

5. Serve the spinach and sweet potatoes immediately with the roasted fish fillets and yoghurt.

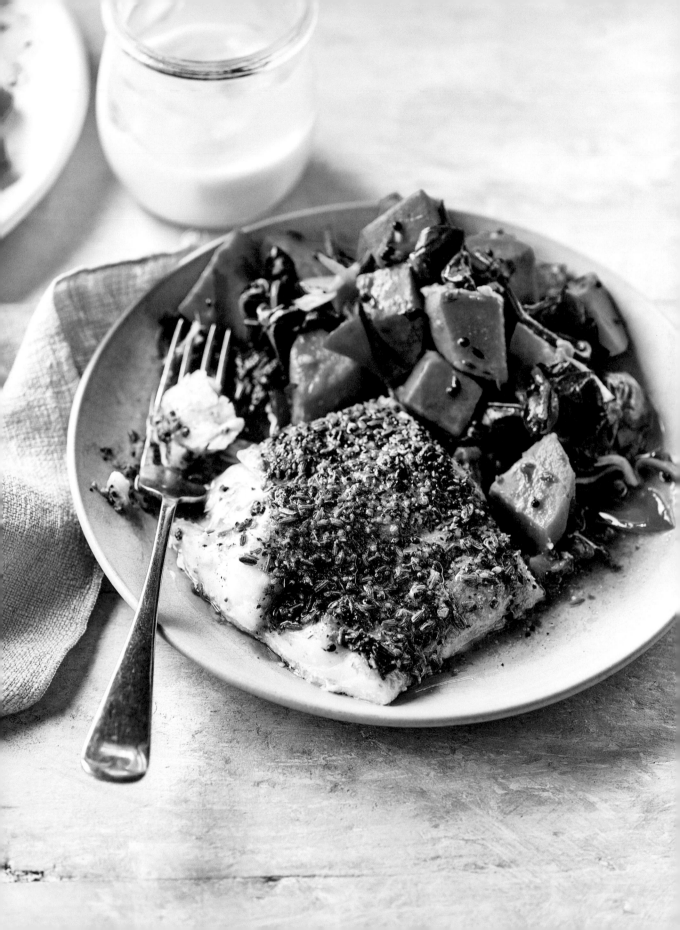

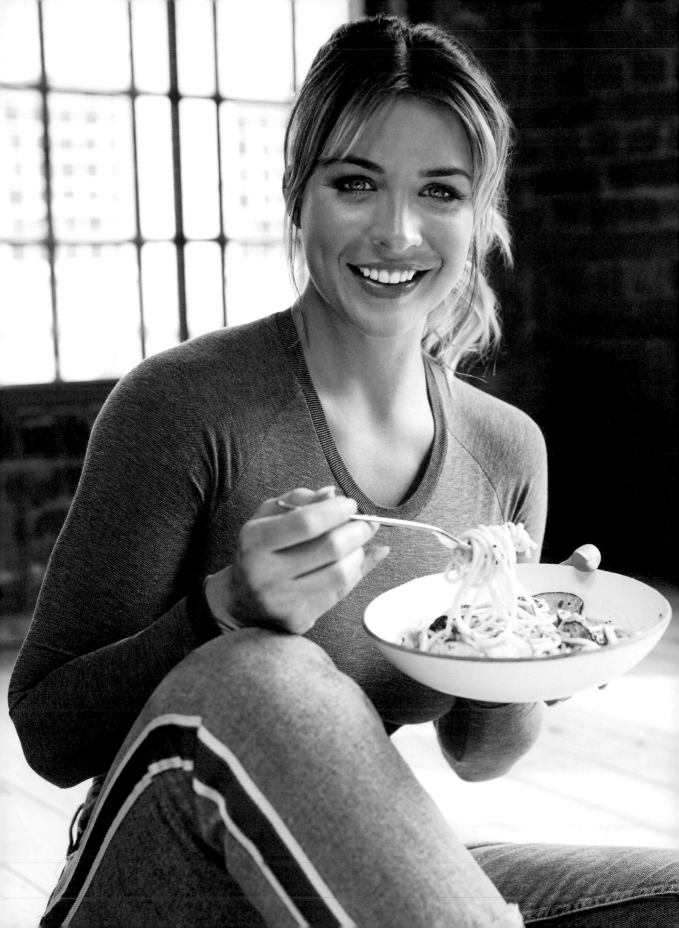

Salmon & Courgette Spaghetti

640kcals PER SERVING | SERVES 2 | PREP TIME 5 MIN | COOKING TIME 20-25 MIN

This recipe is great for making a small amount of salmon go a long way!

200g/7oz spaghetti (dry weight)

1 tbsp olive oil

2 courgettes (zucchini), thinly sliced

125g/4½oz skinned salmon fillet, cubed

4 tbsp white wine

60ml (2fl oz/¼ cup) half-fat crème fraîche

grated zest of 1 lemon and a squeeze of juice

a small bunch of chives, snipped

salt and freshly ground black pepper

1. Cook the spaghetti according to the packet instructions. Drain well and return the pasta to the warm pan.
2. Heat the olive oil in a frying pan (skillet) set over a medium heat, add the courgettes (zucchini) and cook, turning occasionally for 2 minutes. Add the salmon and cook, stirring once or twice, for 2 minutes.
3. Add the wine and cook for 2-3 minutes until it reduces and the salmon is cooked through. Remove from the heat and stir in the crème fraîche, lemon zest and a squeeze of lemon juice. Season to taste with salt and pepper.
4. Add the creamy salmon and courgette to the spaghetti together with the chives and toss everything gently to coat the pasta strands lightly.
5. Divide between two shallow bowls and serve immediately.

Ginger Chicken & Kale Stir Fry

475kcals PER SERVING | SERVES 2 | PREP TIME 10 MIN | COOKING TIME 15 MIN

Ginger and chicken are a match made in taste-bud heaven (don't skimp on the lemongrass).

100g (4oz/scant ½ cup) basmati rice

1 tbsp vegetable or sesame oil

250g/9oz chicken breast fillets, cubed

2 garlic cloves, crushed

2.5cm/1in piece of fresh root ginger, peeled and diced

1 stalk lemongrass, peeled and diced

1 red or green chilli, deseeded and diced

1 red or yellow (bell) pepper, deseeded and thinly sliced

125g/4½oz kale, chopped or shredded

2 tbsp soy sauce

1. Cook the rice according to the packet instructions.
2. Meanwhile, heat the oil in a wok or large, deep frying pan (skillet) set over a medium-high heat. Add the chicken and stir-fry for 5-6 minutes until golden brown all over.
3. Add the garlic, ginger, lemongrass, chilli and sliced (bell) pepper and stir-fry for 2 minutes. Add the kale and cook for about 3 minutes until wilted but still crisp. Stir in the soy sauce.
4. Serve immediately with the cooked rice.

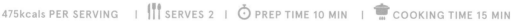 **TIP:** You can use other greens instead of kale – try chopped spring greens or Savoy cabbage or even broccoli florets.

GF

Easy Chicken Korma

610kcals PER SERVING | ⏗ SERVES 2 | ⏱ PREP TIME 10 MIN | 🍲 COOKING TIME 25-30 MIN

People can get intimidated by the thought of making a curry, but this recipe will prove that a home-cooked version can be both easy and really healthy – and will always taste better than one you've ordered in. I use fresh chilli and spices to flavour the korma but you can buy ready-made Korma spice mix or paste if you prefer.

1 tbsp olive or vegetable oil

200g/7oz chicken breast fillets, cubed

½ red onion, thinly sliced

2 garlic cloves, crushed

1 red chilli, diced

1cm/½in piece of fresh root ginger, peeled and finely diced or grated

1 tsp cumin seeds

1 tsp ground coriander

1 tsp garam masala

½ tsp ground turmeric

200ml (7fl oz/generous ¾ cup) canned reduced-fat coconut milk

120ml (4fl oz/½ cup) chicken stock

100g/4oz fine green beans, trimmed and halved

4 tbsp 0% fat Greek yoghurt

100g (4oz/scant ½ cup) basmati rice (dry weight)

FRESH RED ONION CHUTNEY

½ red onion, finely chopped

1 tsp garam masala

a small bunch of coriander (cilantro), chopped

juice of 1 lime

1. Make the fresh red onion chutney: mix all the ingredients together in a bowl and set aside.

2. Heat the oil in a deep frying pan (skillet) set over a medium heat. Add the chicken and onion and cook, stirring occasionally, for 6–8 minutes until the onion is soft and the chicken is golden brown. Stir in the garlic, chilli, ginger and cumin seeds and cook for 2 minutes. Stir in the ground spices and cook for a further 2 minutes.

3. Add the coconut milk and stock and bring to the boil. Reduce the heat, cover the pan and simmer gently for 10–15 minutes until the chicken is cooked through and the sauce is creamy and reduced. Add the beans 5 minutes before the end of cooking. Remove from the heat and stir in the yoghurt.

4. Meanwhile, cook the rice according to the packet instructions.

5. Divide the rice and korma between two serving bowls and serve with the chutney.

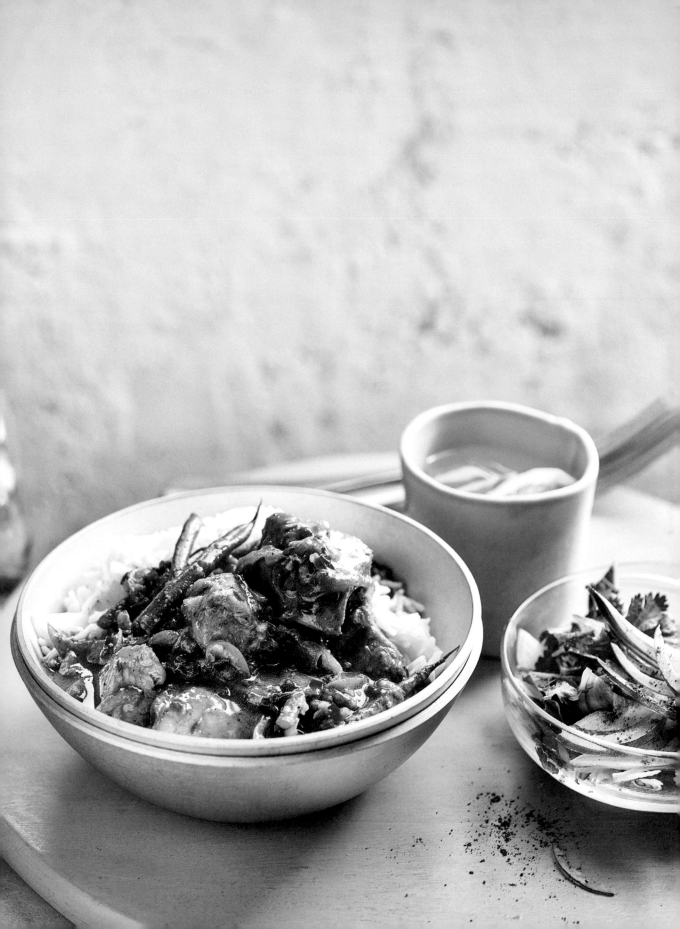

Spring Chicken Risotto

575kcals PER SERVING | ￭￭￭ SERVES 2 | ⏱ PREP TIME 10 MIN | 🍲 COOKING TIME 35-40 MIN

Whatever you do – don't stop stirring! Follow that golden rule when making a risotto and you won't go wrong. You can vary the vegetables by adding broad beans, mangetout, sugar snap peas or baby spinach. Or try stirring in some fresh green pesto before serving.

a small bunch of spring onions (scallions), trimmed and halved

100g/4oz thin or baby asparagus spears, trimmed

100g/4oz shelled peas (or frozen ones)

2 courgettes (zucchini), sliced

420ml (14fl oz/1¾ cups) hot chicken stock

1 tbsp olive oil

1 onion, chopped

125g (4½oz/generous ½ cup) arborio or carnaroli risotto rice (dry weight)

75ml (2½fl oz/generous ¼ cup) white wine or dry vermouth

150g/5oz cooked skinned chicken, shredded

juice of ½ lemon

2 tbsp grated Parmesan cheese

a handful of parsley, chopped

salt and freshly ground black pepper

1. Blanch the spring onions (scallions), asparagus, peas and courgettes (zucchini) in a saucepan of boiling water for 2–3 minutes until just tender. Refresh under cold running water, then drain and set aside.

2. Put the hot chicken stock in pan on the stovetop and keep it simmering over a low heat.

3. Heat the oil in a heavy-based wide frying pan (skillet) or saucepan set over a low–medium heat, add the onion and cook, stirring occasionally, for about 5 minutes until softened but not browned. Stir in the rice and cook for 1–2 minutes, stirring, until it starts to crackle.

4. Pour in the wine or vermouth and cook over a medium heat until it has reduced and almost evaporated. Reduce the heat to a gentle simmer and start adding the hot stock, a ladleful at a time, stirring until each ladleful has been absorbed before adding more.

5. When all or most of the stock has been added and the rice is cooked and tender but not too soft, after 15–20 minutes, gently stir in the chicken, lemon juice and blanched vegetables. Cook for 2 minutes to heat everything through.

6. Take the pan off the heat and stir in the Parmesan and parsley. Season to taste with salt and pepper and leave to rest for 2–3 minutes before serving in shallow bowls.

Pork & Mushroom Pasta Ribbons

610kcals PER SERVING | ¶¶¶ SERVES 2 | ⏱ PREP TIME 40 MIN | 🍲 COOKING TIME 25-30 MIN

You can buy packets of dried mushrooms in almost any supermarket. They're so easy to use and add a wonderfully intense flavour to sauces for pasta.

15g/½oz dried mushrooms (preferably porcini or ceps)

1 tbsp olive oil

200g/7oz pork fillet (tenderloin), trimmed and cut into thin strips

1 small onion, thinly sliced

200g/7oz chestnut mushrooms, sliced

100ml (3½fl oz/scant ½ cup) white wine

200ml (7fl oz/generous ¾ cup) chicken stock

120g (4½oz/½ cup) half-fat crème fraîche

1 tsp wholegrain mustard

grated zest of 1 lemon

200g/7oz pasta ribbons, e.g. tagliatelle or fettuccine (dry weight)

salt and freshly ground black pepper

2 tbsp chopped parsley, to serve

1. Pour some boiling water over the dried mushrooms in a heatproof jug or bowl and leave them to soak for at least 30 minutes. Drain well, reserving the soaking liquid.

2. Heat the oil in a large, deep frying pan (skillet) set over a medium-high heat, add the pork strips and cook for 4-5 minutes until browned all over. Remove and set aside.

3. Add the onion and chestnut mushrooms to the pan and cook, stirring occasionally, until the mushrooms are golden and the onions are soft. Add the wine, turn up the heat and let it bubble away until reduced by at least half.

4. Return the pork to the pan with the drained mushrooms. Add the chicken stock and a little of the reserved mushroom soaking liquid. Stir well and simmer for 10-15 minutes until the pork is cooked and tender and the liquid has reduced. Stir in the crème fraîche, mustard and lemon zest and warm through gently for 2 minutes. Season to taste with salt and pepper.

5. Meanwhile, cook the pasta according to the packet instructions. Drain well and divide between two shallow bowls. Spoon the pork and mushroom sauce over the top and sprinkle with parsley.

 VARIATION:

· Swap the pork for chicken breast fillet strips.

Baked Cod with Chilli & Chickpeas

510kcals PER SERVING | ⦚⦚⦚ SERVES 2 | ⏱ PREP TIME 10 MIN | 🍲 COOKING TIME 15 MIN

I've put cod here, but any thick fish fillets will work just as well in this easy dish – haddock, monkfish or whiting are all good choices, being low in fat and a great source of protein.

2 x 150g/5oz thick cod fillets (with skin)

1 tbsp peeled and grated fresh root ginger

1 red chilli, deseeded and shredded

grated zest and juice of 1 large lime

1 tbsp olive oil, plus extra for brushing

1 red onion, thinly sliced

2 garlic cloves, crushed

400g/14oz canned chickpeas (garbanzo beans), rinsed and drained

200g/7oz spring greens or spinach, washed and shredded

a pinch of dried chilli flakes

salt and freshly ground black pepper

lime wedges, to serve

1. Preheat the oven to 200°C/180°C fan/400°F/gas 6.
2. Place the cod, skin side down, in an oiled roasting pan. Sprinkle the ginger, chilli and lime juice over the fish and season with salt and pepper. Bake in the oven for 15 minutes until the fish is opaque and cooked through.
3. Meanwhile, heat the oil in a frying pan (skillet) set over a medium heat, add the onion and cook, stirring occasionally, for about 8 minutes until softened. Stir in the garlic and cook for 1 minute.
4. Add the chickpeas (garbanzo beans) and greens and cook over a low heat for 2–3 minutes until the greens wilt and the chickpeas are hot. Season with salt and pepper and sprinkle with lime zest and chilli flakes.
5. Serve the chickpeas immediately with the baked cod fillets, with lime wedges for squeezing.

💡 VARIATIONS:

· Use pak choi (bok choy) or Tenderstem broccoli instead of the spring greens or spinach.
· If you don't have lime, substitute lemon.
· Add a shake of soy sauce to the greens just before serving.

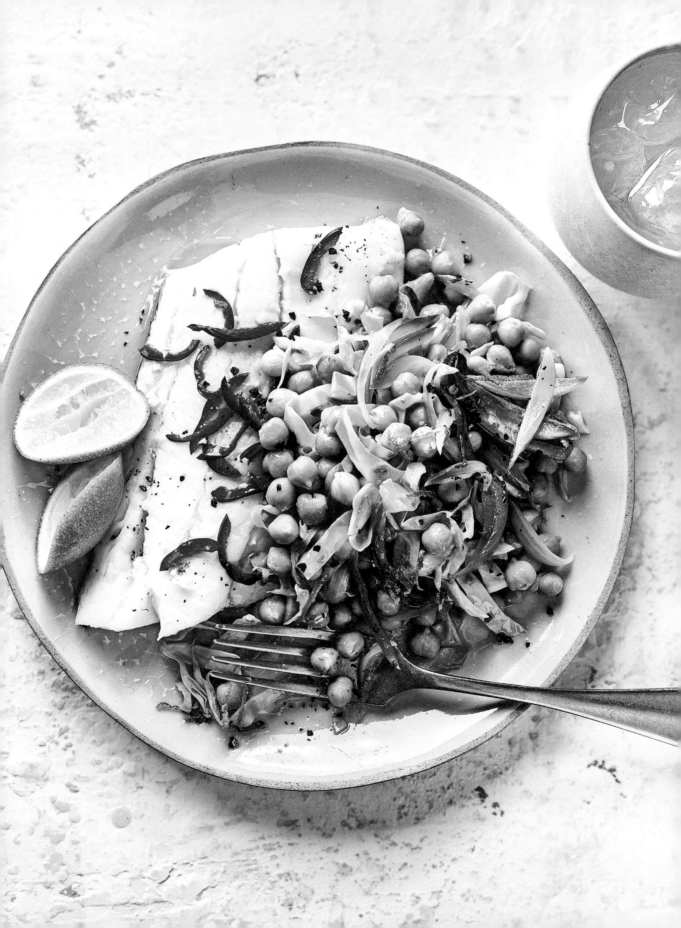

Stewed Beef & Roots with Fruity Parsnip Smash

550kcals PER SERVING | SERVES 4 | PREP TIME 20 MIN | COOKING TIME 3 HRS

There's nothing as satisfying or comforting as a hearty stew and this recipe ticks all the boxes. You need to plan ahead for this one as it takes a few hours to cook, but the results are well worth it. It's got Sunday dinner written all over it.

1 tbsp olive oil

600g/1lb 5oz lean stewing beef, cubed

2 large onions, chopped

2 carrots, sliced

400g/14oz swede (rutabaga), cubed

3 celery sticks, thinly sliced

1 rounded tbsp plain (all-purpose) flour

1.2 litres (2 pints/5 cups) hot beef stock

2 tbsp wholegrain mustard

2 bay leaves

thin strip of orange zest (see Tip)

salt and freshly ground black pepper

a handful of parsley, chopped, to serve

FRUITY PARSNIP SMASH

600g/1lb 5oz parsnips, peeled and cut into chunks

200g/7oz potatoes, peeled and cut into chunks

2 large cooking (green) apples, peeled, cored and thickly sliced

100ml (3½fl oz/scant ½ cup) skimmed, soya or nut milk

25g (1oz/2 tbsp) butter

a pinch of ground nutmeg

salt and freshly ground black pepper

1. Heat the oil in a large heavy-based saucepan or flameproof casserole dish set over a medium–high heat. Add the beef (in batches if necessary) and cook for 6–8 minutes, stirring often, until browned all over. Remove with a slotted spoon and drain on kitchen paper (paper towels).

2. Add the onions, carrots, swede (rutabaga) and celery to the pan. Reduce the heat and cook for 5 minutes, stirring occasionally. Stir in the flour and cook for 1 minute, then stir in the stock and bring to the boil. Reduce the heat to a simmer and add the beef, mustard, bay leaves and strip of orange zest. Season with salt and pepper.

3. Cover the pan and simmer gently over a low heat for 2–2¼ hours or until the vegetables are cooked and the beef is tender and falling apart. Remove and discard the orange zest and bay leaves.

4. Meanwhile, make the fruity parsnip smash: bring a saucepan of water to the boil and add the parsnips, potatoes and apples. Reduce the heat and simmer for 10–12 minutes until tender. Drain well. Return everything to the warm pan and add the milk and butter. Mash with a potato masher until smooth and there are no lumps. Season to taste with nutmeg and salt and pepper.

5. Serve the stew, sprinkled with parsley, with the fruity parsnip smash.

TIP: Use a potato peeler to peel a long strip of zest off an orange.

Spicy Bean & Pumpkin Stew

610kcals PER SERVING | ††† SERVES 4 | ⏱ PREP TIME 15 MIN | 🍲 COOKING TIME 1 HR

This Cajun-style veggie stew is packed with nutrients and makes four servings, so you can cool any leftover portions and keep them in the fridge for another meal, or freeze them for a later date.

2 tbsp coconut or vegetable oil

1 large onion, chopped

3 garlic cloves, crushed

1cm/½in piece of fresh root ginger, peeled and diced

3 red and yellow (bell) peppers, deseeded and cut into chunks

1.3kg/3lb pumpkin, peeled, deseeded and cut into chunks

1 tbsp paprika

1 tsp cayenne

1 tsp dried thyme

150ml (5fl oz/scant ¾ cup) vegetable stock

400ml (14fl oz/1½ cups) canned reduced-fat coconut milk

400g (14oz/2 cups) canned chopped tomatoes

400g (14oz/2 cups) canned kidney beans, rinsed and drained

200g (7oz/scant 1 cup) brown or basmati rice (dry weight)

salt and freshly ground black pepper

TO SERVE

4 tbsp 0% fat Greek yoghurt

a few sprigs of coriander (cilantro), chopped

1. Heat the oil in a large saucepan set over a low heat. Add the onion, garlic, ginger and (bell) peppers and cook, stirring occasionally, for 8–10 minutes until tender and just starting to brown. Add the pumpkin and cook for 2–3 minutes.

2. Stir in the spices and thyme and cook for 1 minute. Add the stock, coconut milk and tomatoes and bring to the boil. Reduce the heat to a gentle simmer and stir in the kidney beans. Cook for about 40 minutes, stirring from time to time, until all the vegetables are really tender and the liquid has reduced. Season to taste with salt and pepper.

3. Meanwhile, cook the rice according to the packet instructions.

4. Divide the rice between 4 serving plates and spoon the stew over the top. Add a spoonful of yoghurt and sprinkle with coriander (cilantro).

💡 VARIATION:

· If you can't get pumpkin, try butternut squash instead.

Cheesy Roots Pie

640kcals PER SERVING | ⊪ SERVES 2 | ⏱ PREP TIME 15 MIN | 🍲 COOKING TIME 30–40 MIN

Is there anything better than reading the words 'cheese' and 'pie' together when you're hungry? No! Nothing can beat it. This pie is cheap, easy to make and full of healthy veg. If you want to add more, or change some of them up, how about peppers, courgettes or even some baby spinach leaves?

1 tbsp olive oil

2 garlic cloves, crushed

1 large leek, trimmed, washed and thickly sliced

200g/7oz chestnut mushrooms, sliced

200g/7oz cherry tomatoes, halved

a handful of parsley, finely chopped

2 tbsp grated Cheddar cheese

MASHED ROOTS

500g/1lb 2oz mixture of sweet potatoes, parsnips, swede (rutabaga) or potatoes, peeled and cubed

15g (½oz/1 tbsp) butter

2 tbsp skimmed milk

4 spring onions (scallions), trimmed and finely chopped

75g (3oz/¾ cup) Cheddar cheese, grated

salt and freshly ground black pepper

1. Preheat the oven to 200°C/180°C fan/400°F/gas 6.
2. Make the mashed roots: put the cubed vegetables into a saucepan of lightly salted water and bring to the boil. Reduce the heat and simmer gently for 10–15 minutes until cooked and tender. Drain well and return to the hot pan. Mash with the butter and milk. Add a good grinding of black pepper and stir in the spring onions (scallions) and Cheddar.
3. Meanwhile, heat the oil in a large frying pan (skillet) set over a low–medium heat, add the garlic and leek and cook, stirring occasionally, for 6–8 minutes until softened. Add the mushrooms and cook for 3–4 minutes until golden. Stir in the tomatoes and cook for 2–3 minutes, squashing them slightly with the back of a wooden spoon. Stir in the parsley.
4. Cover the base of a shallow ovenproof dish with half of the mashed roots, then spoon the cooked vegetables over the top. Cover with the remaining mashed roots and rough up the top with the prongs of a fork. Sprinkle with the grated Cheddar.
5. Bake in the oven for 20–25 minutes until golden brown and crisp on top. Serve immediately.

MAIN MEALS

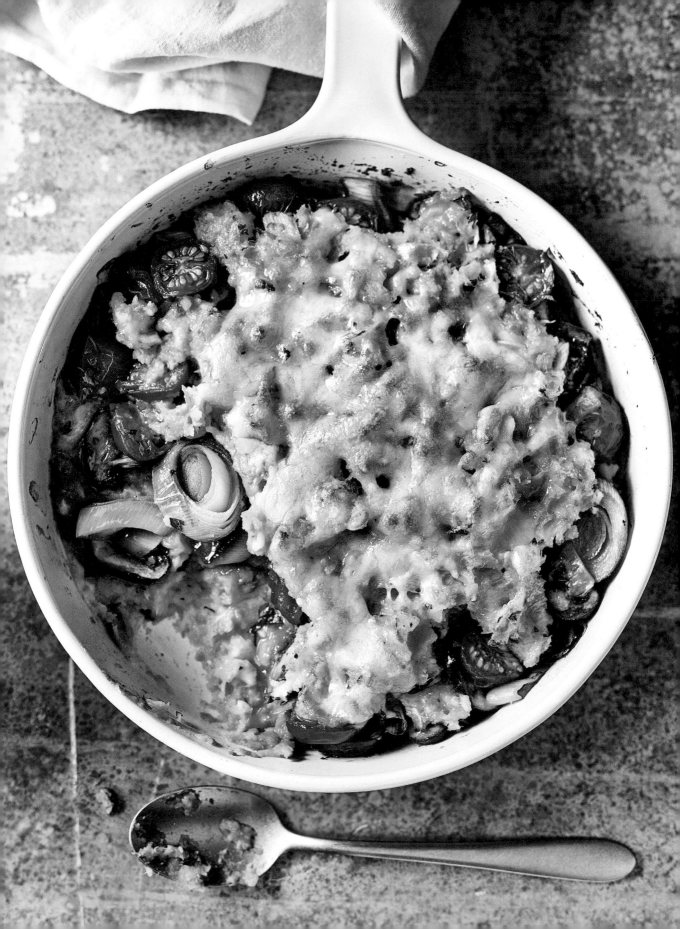

Seafood Risotto

650kcals PER SERVING | ￼ SERVES 2 | ⏱ PREP TIME 10 MIN | ￼ COOKING TIME 35–45 MIN

Seafood is a good source of zinc and selenium, which supports your immune system. For speed and convenience, I use a packet of frozen seafood (fruits de mer) to make this brilliant risotto – it's always worth keeping a spare packet in the freezer ready to defrost for an easy dinner.

1 tbsp olive oil

1 onion, finely chopped

2 garlic cloves, crushed

480ml (16fl oz/2 cups) hot fish or
vegetable stock

a pinch of dried chilli flakes or chilli
powder

125g (4½oz/½ cup) arborio or
carnaroli risotto rice (dry weight)

120ml (4fl oz/½ cup) white wine

a pinch of saffron threads

100g/4oz baby plum tomatoes,
halved

400g/14oz frozen mixed seafood,
e.g. prawns (shrimp), mussels,
squid, scallops, defrosted

juice of 1 lemon

a small bunch of parsley, chopped

salt and freshly ground black pepper

1. Heat the oil in a heavy-based wide saucepan set over a low heat, add the onion and garlic and cook, stirring occasionally, for 8–10 minutes until softened but not browned.

2. Put the hot fish or vegetable stock in saucepan on the stovetop and keep it simmering over a low heat.

3. Stir the chilli and rice into the onions and garlic and cook for 2–3 minutes until the grains are glistening with oil and start crackling. Pour in the wine and turn up the heat. Cook for 2–3 minutes until the liquid has reduced and almost evaporated.

4. Reduce the heat to a gentle simmer and add a ladleful of the hot stock with the saffron and cook gently, stirring, until all the liquid has been absorbed. Add another ladle of stock and continue stirring and adding more in this way until the rice is tender but not too soft.

5. Stir in the tomatoes and seafood. Cook for a few more minutes until the prawns (shrimp) turn pink and the tomatoes start to soften.

6. Remove from the heat and season to taste with salt and pepper. Stir in the lemon juice and parsley. Cover the pan and set aside to rest for 5 minutes before serving.

☀ VARIATION:

· Add some chunks of fresh cod or salmon fillet or stir in a can of white crab meat at the end.

· Swap fresh tomatoes for canned chopped tomatoes.

MAIN MEALS

Cheesy Chicken & Broccoli Bake

575kcals PER SERVING | ꝐꝐꝐ SERVES 2 | ⏱ PREP TIME 15 MIN | 🍲 COOKING TIME 30-40 MIN

A 'bake' might send shivers down the spine of traditional dieters, but ignore them. This cheese sauce is healthier, quicker and easier to make than a traditional one made with flour and butter and it tastes even better, without the added dollop of guilt.

1 tbsp olive oil

1 onion, finely chopped

250g/9oz chicken breast fillets, cut into chunks

300g/10oz broccoli, cut into florets

30g (1oz/generous ½ cup) fresh white breadcrumbs

2 tbsp grated Cheddar or Parmesan cheese

paprika or cayenne pepper, for dusting

CHEESE SAUCE

1 heaped tbsp cornflour (cornstarch)

300ml (½ pint/1¼ cups) skimmed milk

60g (2oz/generous ½ cup) Cheddar cheese, grated

salt and freshly ground black pepper

1. Preheat the oven to 200°C/180°C fan/400°F/gas 6.

2. Heat the oil in a frying pan (skillet) set over a medium heat. Add the onion and cook, stirring occasionally, for 5 minutes, then stir in the chicken and cook for 5–6 minutes, turning the chunks a few times, until cooked through and golden brown. Remove from the pan and transfer to an ovenproof baking dish.

3. Meanwhile, steam or boil the broccoli for 3–4 minutes until just tender. Drain and add to the chicken in the baking dish.

4. Make the cheese sauce: blend the cornflour (cornstarch) in a bowl with a little of the milk to make a smooth paste. Heat the remaining milk in a pan and when it starts to boil, reduce the heat and stir in the cornflour mixture with a wooden spoon. Keep stirring over a low heat until the sauce thickens and becomes glossy and smooth. Remove from the heat and stir in the grated cheese. Season to taste with salt and pepper.

5. Pour the sauce over the chicken and broccoli. Sprinkle the breadcrumbs and grated Cheddar or Parmesan over the top.

6. Bake in the oven for 20–30 minutes until bubbling, crisp and golden brown on top. Dust with paprika or cayenne and serve immediately.

🔆 **TIP:** You can substitute the broccoli for other vegetables. Try cauliflower and add some shredded spinach, kale or spring greens.

Quick & Easy Fish Stew Bowls

450kcals PER SERVING | ￦ SERVES 2 | ⏱ PREP TIME 15 MIN | 🍲 COOKING TIME 25–30 MIN

The saffron in this fish stew recipe is optional, as not all supermarkets stock it, but if you can find it, it's totally worth adding as it gives the stew a lovely subtle flavour and rich golden colour.

1 tbsp olive oil

1 onion, chopped

1 carrot, thickly sliced

1 celery stick, diced

2 garlic cloves, crushed

250g/9oz sweet potatoes, peeled and cubed

420ml (14fl oz/1¾ cups) hot fish or vegetable stock

200g/7oz tomatoes, roughly chopped

a pinch of dried chilli flakes

a pinch of saffron strands or powdered saffron (optional)

1 bay leaf

strip of orange zest

200g/7oz thick cod or haddock fillet (frozen and defrosted or fresh), skinned and cut into chunks

200g/7oz frozen shelled raw king prawns (jumbo shrimp), defrosted

a dash of lemon or orange juice

a handful of parsley or dill, chopped

salt and freshly ground black pepper

1. Heat the oil in a large saucepan set over a low–medium heat, add the onion, carrot, celery and garlic and cook, stirring occasionally, for 5 minutes. Add the cubed sweet potatoes and cook for 3 minutes.

2. Add the hot stock, tomatoes, chilli flakes, saffron (if using), bay leaf and orange zest strip. Bring to the boil, then reduce the heat and simmer gently for 10 minutes.

3. Add the fish and simmer for 5 minutes, then stir in the prawns (shrimp) and cook for another 3 minutes or so until they turn pink. The vegetables should be tender and the cod should be opaque and thoroughly cooked.

4. Add a little lemon or orange juice and some salt and pepper to taste. Remove the bay leaf and stir in the chopped herbs. Ladle into two shallow bowls to serve.

MAIN MEALS

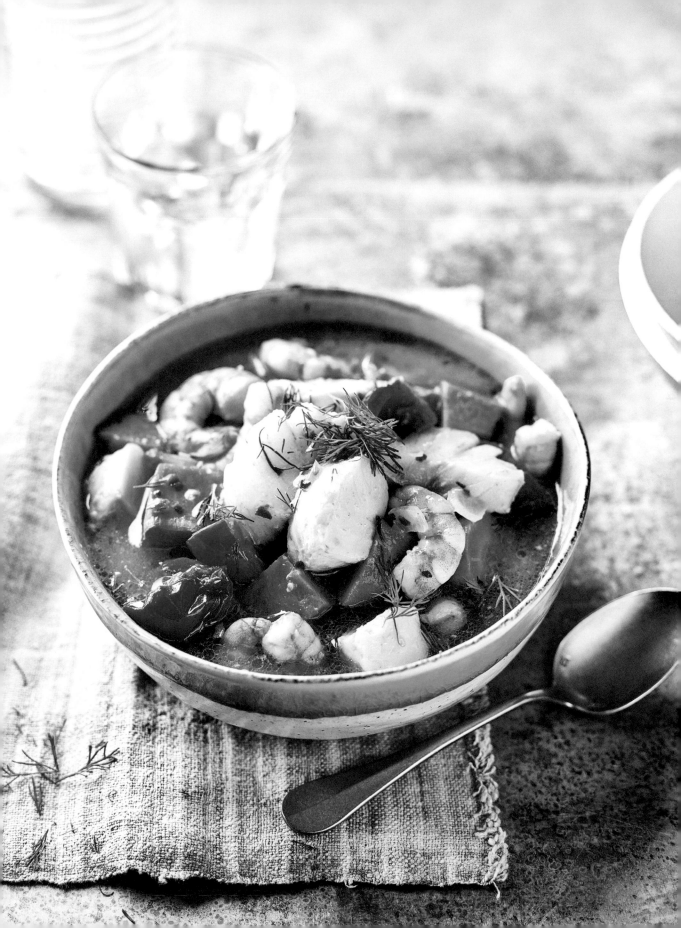

Chicken Cacciatore with Herby Smashed Beans

610kcals PER SERVING | ▌▌▌ SERVES 4 | ⏱ PREP TIME 15 MIN | 🍲 COOKING TIME 1 HR

This recipe is sure to impress at a dinner party, or for a romantic evening in (maybe lay off the garlic in that case though...), as it tastes rich and looks gorgeous, yet is low in calories.

4 bone-in chicken thighs, skinned
1 tbsp plain (all-purpose) flour
1 tbsp olive oil
6 garlic cloves, crushed
2 carrots, cut into small chunks
200g/7oz mushrooms, halved or
   quartered
a few sprigs of rosemary
240ml (8fl oz/1 cup) hot chicken
   stock
2 tbsp low-fat crème fraîche
salt and freshly ground black pepper

HERBY SMASHED BEANS
1 tbsp olive oil
1 onion, finely chopped
100g/4oz baby spinach leaves
400g (14oz/2 cups) canned cannellini
   beans, rinsed and drained
grated zest of 1 lemon
a handful of parsley, finely chopped

1. Dust the chicken lightly with the flour. Heat the oil in a large, deep, heavy-based frying pan (skillet) or saucepan set over a medium heat. Add the chicken and cook, turning occasionally, for about 5 minutes until golden brown all over.

2. Add the garlic, carrots and mushrooms and cook for 5 minutes, then add the rosemary and stock. Cover and simmer gently for 45 minutes until the chicken is cooked through and the liquid has reduced. Stir in the crème fraîche and season to taste with salt and pepper.

3. Meanwhile, make the herby smashed beans: heat the oil in a small saucepan set over a low heat, add the onion and cook for 10 minutes until really tender. Add the spinach and cook for 1–2 minutes until it wilts. Blitz the onion and spinach with the beans, lemon zest and parsley in a blender or food processor until you have a thick purée. Season to taste.

4. Serve the chicken and vegetables in the creamy sauce with the herby smashed beans.

Chicken & Spring Vegetable Pot Roast

550kcals PER SERVING | SERVES 4 | PREP TIME 10 MIN | COOKING TIME 1 HR 20 MIN

A pot roast is so easy: just put everything into a pan and leave it to cook away while you do something else (like a workout, perhaps?) … and there's hardly anything to wash up! If you don't want to use cider for calorie reasons, just double the amount of chicken stock.

1 red onion, cut into wedges

2 leeks, trimmed, washed and thickly sliced

500g/1lb 2oz Chantenay or baby carrots, trimmed and left whole or halved

3 garlic cloves, crushed

4 tomatoes, skinned and chopped

1 x 1.3kg/3lb whole chicken

300ml (½ pint/1¼ cups) chicken stock

300ml (½ pint/1¼ cups) dry cider

1 bay leaf

800g/1¾lb new potatoes, halved or cut into chunks

2 courgettes (zucchini), thickly sliced

a large handful of parsley, finely chopped

salt and freshly ground black pepper

1. Put the red onion, leeks, carrots, garlic and tomatoes in a large heavy-based saucepan or flameproof casserole dish with a lid.
2. Pat the chicken dry with kitchen paper (paper towels). Remove any fat remaining inside and peel away and discard as much skin as possible. Season the flesh with salt and pepper and place the chicken, breast side down, in the pan with the vegetables.
3. Pour the stock and cider over the top, add the bay leaf and cover with a lid. Set over a high heat until the liquid starts to boil, then reduce the heat to a simmer and cook gently for 30 minutes.
4. Turn the chicken over, so it's breast side up, and add the potatoes. Cover the pan and cook gently for about 45 minutes until everything is thoroughly cooked. To test whether the chicken is done, insert a thin skewer or knife behind the thigh – if the juices run clear, it's ready. Add the courgettes (zucchini) about 10 minutes before the end of the cooking time. Fish out the bay leaf and stir in the parsley.
5. Remove the chicken and carve it into portions. Divide them between four serving plates with the vegetables and pan juices and serve immediately.

Cheesy Pumpkin Bake

490kcals PER SERVING | ☳ SERVES 4 | ⏱ PREP TIME 10 MIN | 🍲 COOKING TIME 45 MIN

This recipe makes use of my go-to half-fat crème fraîche as it's less rich and cloying than the full-fat sort, and healthier too of course. Serve with a fresh salad.

500g/1lb 2oz pumpkin, peeled, deseeded and cut into chunks
a few sprigs of thyme, leaves stripped
2 tsp cumin seeds
120ml (4fl oz/½ cup) vegetable stock
60g (2oz/¼ cup) half-fat crème fraîche
100g/4oz soft goat's cheese, e.g. chèvre, crumbled
2 tbsp pumpkin and/or sunflower seeds
25g (1oz/½ cup) fresh white breadcrumbs
salt and freshly ground black pepper

TOMATO SAUCE
1 tbsp olive oil
1 red onion, finely chopped
2 garlic cloves, crushed
400g (14oz/2 cups) canned chopped tomatoes
a few drops of balsamic vinegar

1. Preheat the oven to 180°C/160°C fan/350°F/gas 4.
2. Put the pumpkin into a large shallow ovenproof dish and sprinkle with the thyme leaves and cumin seeds. Season with black pepper and pour the stock over the top. Bake in the oven for about 25 minutes until just tender but not too soft.
3. Meanwhile, make the tomato sauce: heat the oil in a frying pan (skillet) set over a low heat, add the onion and garlic and cook, stirring occasionally, for 10 minutes until soft. Add the tomatoes and simmer gently for 10 minutes until the sauce reduces and thickens. Add the balsamic vinegar and season to taste with salt and pepper.
4. Spoon the tomato sauce over the pumpkin and dot the top with spoonfuls of crème fraîche and the goat's cheese. Scatter the seeds and breadcrumbs over the top.
5. Bake in the oven for 15 minutes or until the topping is crisp and golden and the sauce is bubbling, then serve.

💡 VARIATIONS:
· Use butternut squash or sweet potato when pumpkin is not in season.
· Sprinkle pine nuts over the top with the seeds and breadcrumbs.

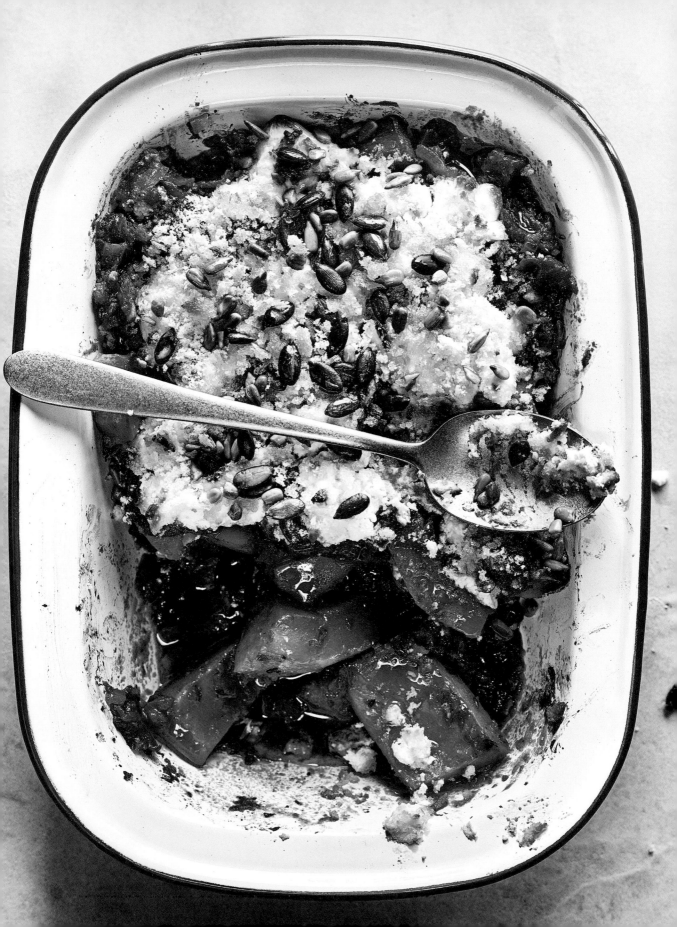

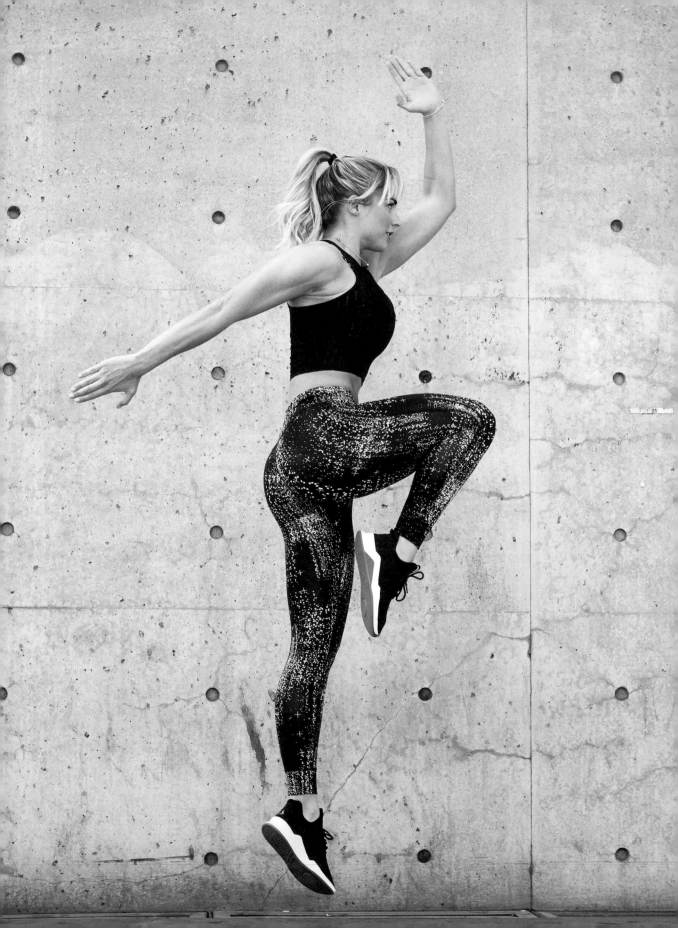

TRAINING

THE 12-WEEK FAT-LOSS TRAINING PLAN

This plan, designed at Ultimate Performance gyms, is split into three different training phases of four weeks each (so 12 weeks altogether, maths fans), which get harder as you progress. For best results, every week you should aim to complete four workout sessions – two HIIT workouts (High Intensity Interval Training) and two weights workouts – while also maintaining a healthy diet (see pages 44-49).

The plan in a nutshell

You should do each phase for four weeks before moving onto the next, and in each phase you'll find four different workouts to choose from: two HIIT routines, one gym-based and one home-based; and two weight routines, again, one gym-based and one home-based. I'm hoping you'll mix it up and do a bit of both, as I really think the camaraderie you'll find in a gym will be motivating, plus you'll have more options when it comes to the weights available to use (unless you happen to have a fully-equipped gym in your house, in which case, congrats!). It's totally up to you, of course, but the choice is there. All of the routines have been carefully created to deliver the same level of results if completed fully, so whether you mix it up, stay at home or stay in the gym, you won't miss out on losing fat and getting lean. See opposite for an example of what a week should look like.

As I said, four workouts a week will deliver you the best results. However, if you can only manage two or three yet stay consistent with your diet, you'll still get there, it may just take a little longer. But that's the joy of this plan. As I've reiterated throughout, while this is a '12-week Fat-loss Plan', there's actually no end date, no cut-off. Once you've got into the groove, it'll become part of your life and so will roll on indefinitely. Don't put yourself under unnecessary pressure if your life is crazy busy – truly commit to doing the best you can, and you'll still reap the rewards.

Monday	Weight training session (home or gym)
Tuesday	HIIT training session (home or gym)
Wednesday	REST DAY
Thursday	Weight training session (home or gym)
Friday	HIIT training session (home or gym)
Saturday	REST DAY (but do a 30-min walk outside)
Sunday	REST DAY

There's a method to the madness

Please do the exercises in each session in the order in which they're presented. Each workout has been designed according to what's called 'stimulation and adaptation'. That means the right muscles are activated and prepped as you go along so you work each muscle to its best advantage, rather than using them 'cold' (and potentially injuring yourself) by jumping from one exercise to the next.

Using your body weight as a tool

The weight-based training programmes have been designed to target the whole body, while paying particular attention to problematic areas for women (see page 164). You'll notice that some of the exercises in these specific sessions don't mention using any free weights (i.e. dumbbells, kettlebells or barbells) or machines. This isn't a mistake! It's because one of the most effective means of strength training is working against your own body weight. When doing press-ups, for example, your body weight acts as the 'load' you're lifting.

Sometimes less is more (or just as much)

Some workouts contain fewer individual exercises than others. This is no indication of difficulty or effectiveness within a phase. Each session should last no longer than 35 minutes, and each has been calculated on the basis of time and effectiveness. You'll soon see that you can be just as shattered working through three exercises as you can be working through eight!

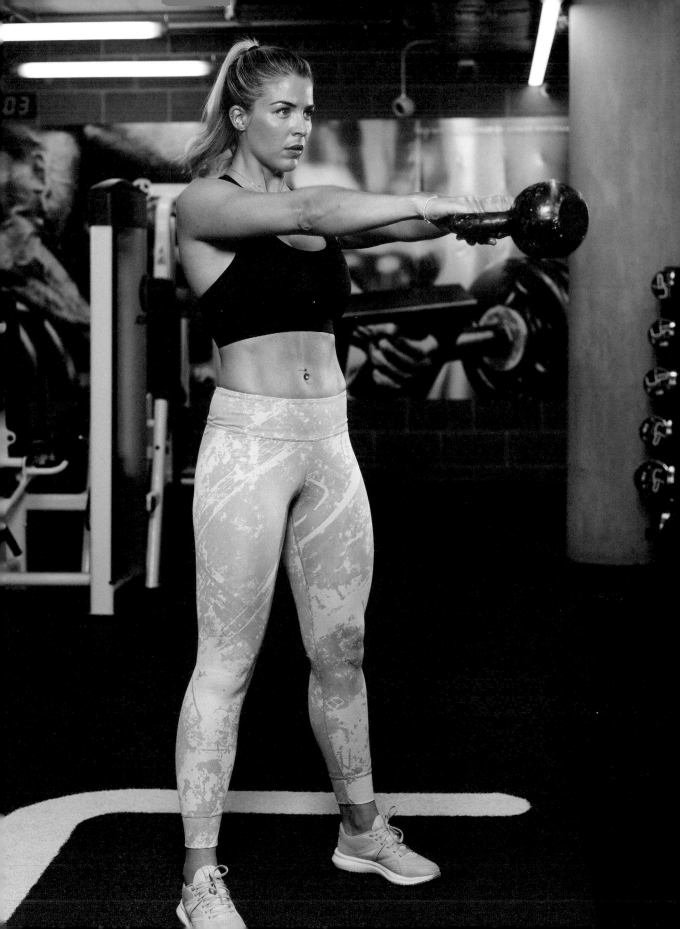

What is HIIT and LISS?

HIIT (High Intensity Interval Training) is short bursts of cardio, performed at 100% of your capacity, followed by short periods of low (or no) exercise as part of your recovery. It's an extremely effective mode of training to achieve greater fat loss over a shorter period of time. It raises your heart rate fast and your body continues to burn fat even after you've finished exercising.

In Phase 2 you'll also come across LISS (Low Intensity Steady State). This is the opposite of HIIT, in that it's low intensity cardio performed at the same pace for a set amount of time. You'll be expending energy and getting a workout while putting less strain on the body, plus it helps to aid recovery.

Why the plan works

A mixture of cardio and weight training is the only way to achieve a sculpted body. Cardio alone cannot produce the muscle toning and sculpting typical of a lean look. As I mentioned at the start of the book, when I was just plodding along for half an hour on a treadmill every day I lost weight, but didn't look toned or feel great (my diet was crap too!). The only way to get truly lean is to do both as the body requires 'overload' to adapt and change.

What is overload?

Overload is when muscles are forced to overcome a resistance they have not experienced before. In simple terms: you need to make your muscles work harder so they adapt to cope, i.e. so they get bigger, stronger and more toned. If you're a beginner, pretty much everything you lift will be overload (and your body weight definitely will be). When you get more advanced you'll need to increase your reps, sets or weight load to keep pushing and making progress. That's why this plan develops and gets tougher as you move through the different phases.

Remember: don't fear weights!

Words like 'overload' and 'bigger muscles' can send shivers down the spine of lots of women, but remember what I said at the start: you will never look 'manly' by weight training; you don't have enough testosterone! What you will do is firm up your body in all the right places.

Lifting weights when combined with cardio will help you torch body fat, improve general strength, help prevent against injury, and, most importantly, it can make you happier and less stressed. Exercise not only releases feel-good endorphins into your system (pleasure-releasing chemicals that also block pain), but it has been proven to help with depression and anxiety. Plus, it just feels great having achieved something you set out to do.

The science bit

Women are built differently to men. That's just a fact. As such, we have different 'problem' areas. For us, these tend to be our glutes (bum), upper thighs and triceps (bingo wings). This is where we store most of our body fat; typically these are the first places we gain weight and the last places we lose it from. Great, huh. Why? Because those areas contain more of the fat receptors (alpha-2) that hinder fat-burning rather than accelerate it. For this reason, many of the exercises in this plan specifically target those areas as they'll need more work, while still training the whole body.

How to get the most out of the plan

1. Always warm up and cool down before each session

It's essential to warm the body up effectively before you start a training session, whether it's HIIT or weight-based. What you do just before you train can have a huge impact on what you get out of the sessions. Most people prepare for a training session by just doing some static stretching and light cardio, neither of which is ideal.

The most effective warm-up is called a 'dynamic pre-mobility routine', which will help mobilise the hips, activate the glutes and open up the chest area. The majority of us spend too much time sitting down, either due to work or because *Blue Planet*'s on, and this can lead to muscle tightness, a rounded back and a sore lower back. The warm-up routine on page 172 will improve these issues as well as physically prepare you for your workout. The cool-down routine on page 176 should be completed at the end of your session. This is the best time for static stretches and should take no longer than three to five minutes.

2. Good form versus bad form

You'll often hear personal trainers bang on about 'good form'. They're not talking about politeness or cleaning down the equipment, they're talking about technique. Good form is fully focusing on the exercise at hand and following the instructions to the letter. Having a wonky spine or locked legs when you shouldn't could lead to serious injury, so whether you're doing HIIT or weights, make sure you focus on the working muscle, follow the instructions, and control your tempo.

Tempo refers to the speed at which a movement is done. Using a controlled tempo will improve your body awareness, improve joint stability in and around the working muscle, improve connective tissue strength and engage the muscle more effectively, leading to better tone. Speeding up to get to the end will not only be a wasted effort, but could lead to injury. Do everything in a controlled, careful manner and you'll see better results.

3. Fully loaded

The term 'load' refers to the amount of weight you should be lifting for the exercise prescribed. It's impossible for me or anyone to be able to tell you what weight is right for you as we're all different, however below is an effective guide to get started:

Unless the exercise is a specific body weight exercise then start by using whatever weights you think are about right and use this rep range equation: if your target rep range is 10–15, give yourself a 5-rep range parameter. This means if you can't get to 10 reps without failing, the load is too heavy; if you can get to 15+ reps without failing, the load is too light. Never sacrifice form for weight load. If you can't maintain technique throughout a whole set, drop the weight until you can. Always work to the rep range! You may even need to alter weights between sets as you fatigue.

Make sure you do a warm-up set of roughly half your intended load before you officially start to get the muscles firing and joints moving.

Some days you will be stronger than others for loads of reasons. Accept this and work as hard as you can that day. Don't beat yourself up about it – but equally, make sure you're listening to your body, not your head (see Commandment 5 on page 37)!

4. Be aware of DOMS (Delayed Onset Muscle Soreness)

DOMS is the official name for that aching that hits the next morning after a good workout. The ache that makes you walk like a cowboy and gasp as you try to put on your socks. It's most pronounced when you introduce a new training routine, a new activity or increase the intensity or volume of your normal workout. It's the result of micro-tears in the muscle fibres that occur when they're strained. That sounds bad, but it's not. It's just the natural process of your muscles being tested. Yeah, it hurts and it can last for several days, but training with DOMS won't result in further damage, and once your body gets used to your new regimen, the DOMS will reduce. That doesn't mean your workout is less effective, it means your muscles are getting stronger! (Don't judge the quality of a workout on the aches you feel afterwards.) There's no way to prevent DOMS, but regular massages, Epsom salt baths and foam rolling post-training can all help.

DOMS is absolutely not the same as an injury – please be aware of the difference. Any short or sharp pains should be investigated, as should any soreness that lasts for more than seven days.

5. Don't ignore the rest days

You're on fire. You've nailed four workouts already and it's only Friday. You're due three rest days, but why bother when you feel this good? BECAUSE YOU HAVE TO. When we exercise, we're inducing changes in the body that include:
- Muscle tissue breakdown
- Depletion of energy stores (muscle glycogen)
- Fluid loss

We're challenging our cardiovascular and musculoskeletal systems, as well as the central nervous system. We're making our body do things it's not used to doing. Even when it is used to doing it, it's not a machine. It still needs time to rest and recuperate. You can't just keep going and going. You will get tired and run-down and will eventually undo all your good work.

Rest days allow our bodies to replenish their energy stores and for muscle tissue to repair itself. Without sufficient time for repair and replenishment, our bodies will, quite simply, work themselves ragged, which can lead to the dangerous state of over-training, which is rare, but not impossible. Far more probable though is you'll just feel knackered and will be unable to continue.

6. Worship at the temple of sleep

Ah, sleep. Magical, wonderful sleep. Isn't it funny how you spend your whole childhood wishing you could stay up late and your whole adulthood wishing someone would just send you to bed?

Sleep is an integral part of this plan. When it comes to achieving your fitness goals, never underestimate the importance of a good night's sleep. Sleep is when the body rests and recovers from the exertions of the previous day, and also prepares for the day ahead. Sleep deprivation will affect you on so many levels, not least messing with the body's levels of leptin and gherlin, the hormones that monitor appetite. A lack of sleep can leave you feeling hungrier and unable to recognise when you're full. It will also affect your energy levels, making you feel sluggish, both physically and mentally. This will not only make you less inclined to work out, but will hinder your recovery time after training. A lack of motivation will make you more likely to skip working out altogether or to do it half-arsed, which will make you feel guilty.

Lots of things can affect our ability to sleep. There are lots of sleep books and apps available that can help you to tackle common sleep issues and to monitor the sleep that you are getting. The good news is that exercising more and eating well will both help you to get to sleep quicker and sleep more soundly through the night. You'll notice this within a month if you keep to the plan.

Here are a few things you can do to help that process:
· No caffeine at least eight hours before bed.
· No alcohol three hours before bed.
· No 'blue light' activity one hour before bed – so no looking at screens that emit 'blue light' (the kind of light that decreases melatonin, the sleepy hormone, in your body). This means no phone, TV or laptop. Read a book, listen to music or have a bath instead.
· Try going to bed and getting up at the same time every day, including weekends. This will help reduce the possibility of 'social jet lag' (when your sleeping patterns are so irregular your body doesn't recognise when to sleep).
· Magnesium supplements can help, as can eating starch-based carbs as part of your last meal of the day (for example, sweet potato, white rice or porridge oats).

7. Keep up your other activities

If you enjoy playing tennis, play tennis! If you love swimming, don't miss out. Just listen to your body and don't risk burn-out, so perhaps swap this other activity for one of your HIIT workouts or do it at half the energy expenditure you usually would (i.e. only play one set of tennis, or one half of a football game.)

Also, on rest days, I strongly suggest you buy yourself a pedometer or fitness tracker and aim to accomplish 8,000 to 10,000 steps a day. Walking 10,000 steps isn't HIIT or strength training. It's a very mellow form of LISS and so won't wear you out and really will help you to reach your goals. If you've never monitored them before, 10,000 steps is actually much more than you probably think, so if you find you're a long way off this target in the beginning, aim to increase your steps each week by a minimum of 500. You can do this by simply getting off the bus a stop earlier on your way to work, taking the stairs rather than the lift or parking further away from the shops when you go shopping.

It's simple – the more you move, the more body fat you'll lose.

8. Track your progress

It's vitally important to track your progress throughout this process. Tracking is proven to increase motivation and decrease any 'Oh, screw it' thoughts. Knowing you're going to have to write down 'scoffed entire carrot cake' really will make you less likely to scoff it. Actually watching a pedometer crank up has been proven to make people walk a little bit further. Plus, knowing you're going to have to stand nearly naked in front of a mirror to take a progress photo (see next section) will make you far less likely to think, 'I'll have that extra glass of wine and skip my workout' the day before.

The best way to track your progress is by doing the weekly reviews listed below.

Snap weekly progress photos
You see yourself every day which makes it extremely difficult for you to fully appreciate any changes occurring. You might think nothing's happened and then see a friend for the first time in months and their mouth will fall open at the difference (it's really amazing when that happens, by the way). This is why photos are both a great way to motivate yourself and also to get a reality check. (It's also common not to realise how far things have gone wrong until we see pictures and think, 'God, is that really what I look like?')

One day a week (Mondays make sense) take a progress photo in your underwear first thing before you've had anything to eat or drink. Take the photos in the same room (one with good light) each week, and don't get self-conscious about it. These photos are for you and you only. You'll be so glad you took them a month into the plan, trust me.

Get out the tape measure
Measure your bust, hips, waist, mid-thighs and upper arms and jot down the results once a week. As I've already mentioned, your weight means nothing on this plan, but your measurements will change. So while you may have actually put on weight on the scales, you'll have lost inches around your hips.

Notice how your clothes fit

A simple but effective way to know you're making progress is to assess how your clothes fit. If those jeans are starting to hang a bit lower off your waist you know you're doing good.

Monitor your mood

How you feel emotionally is one of the most important things to track throughout this whole process, as it'll have the most influence on your desire and determination to see the plan through. Your mood will affect how hard you train, if you train at all, and how rigorously you stick to eating well. If you're feeling low and unmotivated about how things are going, you need to investigate why. This plan demands sacrifices and if it's impacting on work, family, sleep or your overall health perhaps you're pushing it too hard and can relax a bit. Equally, if you're finding no change happening, are you really throwing your all into it? Or are other things happening in your life that are clouding how you feel about this? Often if we're stressed or anxious, it's simple to point the finger at something obvious and, as this plan will have changed things for you and will be tough going at times, it's an easy target.

The table on the opposite page will help to monitor your mood, so you can start noticing patterns (details on filling it out can be found on page 40). You'll be able to see how feeling low affects your behaviour (i.e. whether you then skip training and eat badly), so you can watch out for it. It'll also prove that how you feel before exercising ('I can't be arsed'), bears absolutely no resemblance to how you'll feel afterwards ('I feel proud and energised'). Here's a fact: I have never ever regretted working out. Not once in my whole life. I have, however, regretted not working out. See for yourself. Start monitoring how your mood affects your training and vice versa. And remember, change doesn't happen overnight. This plan is 12 weeks long for a reason. It will take that long to get on the path to a total life overhaul. Keep with it; have faith both in it and yourself. This works.

Terminology

If you are new to the gym or to using weights, you might find some of the terminology confusing at first. Lots of terms are shortened for ease, so here you'll find a handy list of what's what:

DB	=	Dumbbell
KB	=	Kettlebell
ALT	=	Alternating (as in, you alternate sides)
RDL	=	Romanian Deadlift
AMRAP	=	As Many Reps As Possible (keep going until you start to lose form)

Daily motivation table

Draw this table into your notebook and fill it out each morning and evening. It may sound like a drag, but trust me, it'll be worth it. It'll keep you honest about how much you're investing in the plan (and whether you need to up your game) and you'll be able to see how, when you really throw yourself into it, it'll seriously affect your mood for the better. Use this in conjunction with the My Fitness First app to monitor what you're eating, or alternatively, fill in the 'breakfast', 'lunch', 'dinner' and 'snack' columns (see below) so it's all on one table.

I have filled in a couple of examples to show you what I mean.

Date	HOW I FEEL – AM (both physically and mentally)	WORKOUT	BREAKFAST	LUNCH	DINNER	SNACK	HOW I FEEL – PM (both physically and mentally)
02.01.19	Body: Tired Mind: Determined	Home Weights Workout	Green French Toast	Chicken Laksa Bowl	Sweet Potato Jackets with Veggie Chilli	Spicy Roasted Chickpeas	Body: Achy Mind: Proud
03.01.19	Body: Strong Mind: Positive	Gym HIIT	Green Breakfast Smoothie	Chicken & Hummus Wraps	Veggie Burgers	Quick Green Hummus with Oatcakes	Body: Exhausted Mind: Anxious about big work day tomorrow
04.01.19	Body: Nauseous, fidgety Mind: Anxious, worried, insecure	REST DAY	White toast with peanut butter	Packaged ham and cheese sandwich	Pizza	Tortillas and dip	Body: Bloated and uncomfortable Mind: Relieved the day is over but guilty about messing up the plan
05.01.19	Body: Bloated, heavy Mind: Slow after a bad night's sleep	Half-hearted Home Weights Workout	Baked Greek Eggs	Chicken & Aubergine Stacks	Cheesy Roots Pie	Santorini Fava Dip	Body: Better after eating well Mind: Determined to change things up tomorrow
06.01.19	Body: Well rested Mind: Relaxed, confident	Gym HIIT	Eggs & Mushroom Cups	Steak with Paprika Avocado Dip	Stir-fried Crispy Tofu & Vegetables	Chia Seed Pudding	Body: Strong, fit Mind: Looking forward to tomorrow

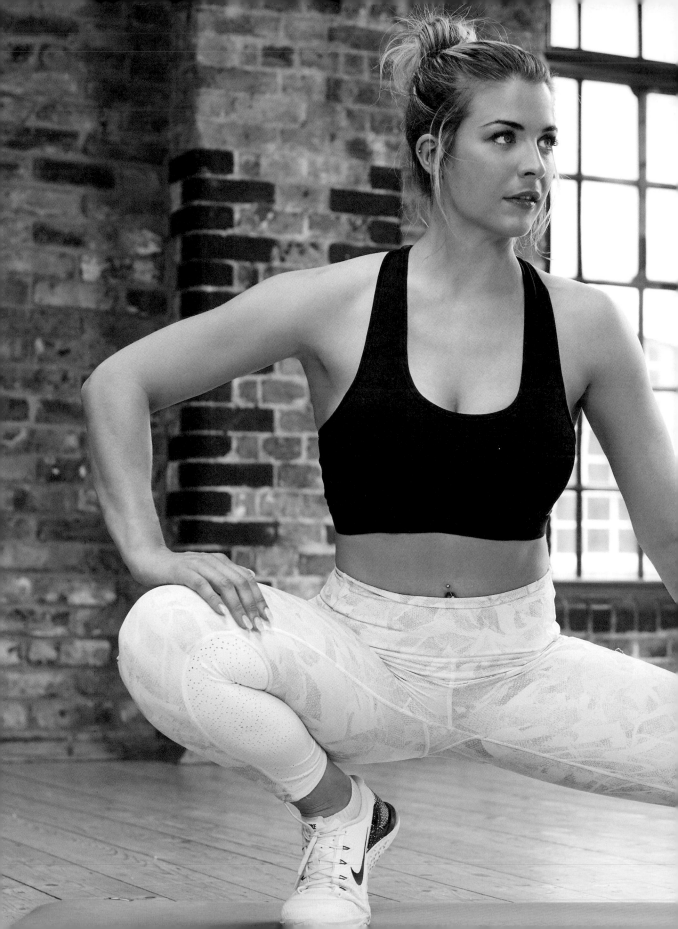

WARM-UP/ COOL-DOWN

YOUR WARM-UP

Both the warm-up and cool-down should take a maximum of five minutes and be completed before every workout in each phase, except for the Phase 2 Gym HIIT section (see notes on page 212).

Exercise	Sets	Reps or Time	Target Area
Hip Flexors Side Step	1	10 per side	Hips
Cat to Dog	1	10	Pelvis
Thoracic Spine 90-90	1	10 per side	Upper Body
Glute Bridges	1	10	Glute Activation
Hamstring Roll	1	10	Hamstrings
Pole or Wall Squat	1	5	Hips & Ankles

 SETS   REPS / TIME

HIP FLEXORS SIDE STEP

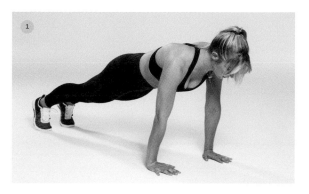

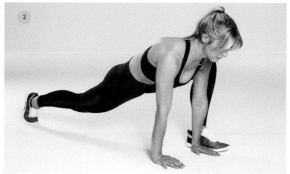

1. Get into a prone position on the floor, supporting your weight through your hands and toes.
2. Bring your left leg round towards your left hand, placing the whole foot on the floor. From here allow the hips to drop down towards the ground to increase the stretch. Pause for a second and then repeat on the other side, alternating between reps.

 1

🕐 10 PER SIDE

CAT TO DOG

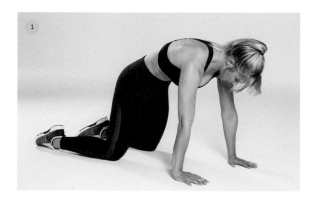

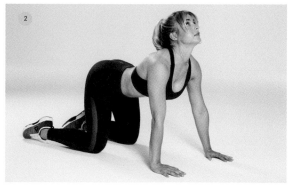

 1

🕐 10

1. Place your hands and knees on the ground. Make sure there is an equal amount of weight placed across the points of contact with the ground. In a smooth movement arch your back up towards the ceiling, sucking your stomach in and tucking your chin into your chest.

2. Once you have flexed as far as you can, arch the other way, lifting your head up, looking towards the ceiling, squeezing your shoulder blades together and allowing the stomach to drop towards the ground. Keep repeating this process for the set reps.

THORACIC SPINE 90-90

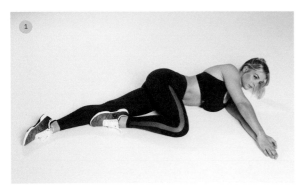

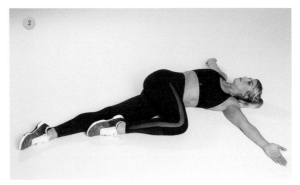

1. Lie on your side with your top hip bent at 90-degrees and your knee resting on the floor or on a foam roller. Actively push this knee down and maintain this throughout to lock your lower back in place. Extend your arm nearest the floor to touch the ground for support.
2. Turn your torso and raise your upper arm so that your upper shoulder is near or touching the floor. Over time, your range during this stretch will improve dramatically.

 1

 10 PER SIDE

GLUTE BRIDGE

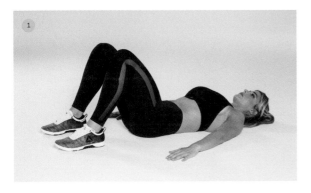

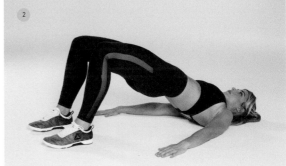

1

10

1. Begin by lying on your back with knees bent and feet flat on the ground, hip-width apart.
2. Lift your hips towards the ceiling, driving your weight through the heels and squeezing the glutes at the top. Don't arch your lower back. Hold for a second at the top, continuing to

squeeze the glutes and making sure your body is in a straight line from the knees to the shoulders.
3. Slowly lower yourself back down to the starting position, rolling your spine down from the top to bottom as you do. Repeat.

HAMSTRING ROLL

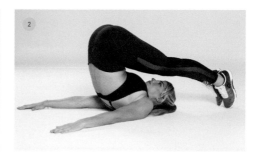

 1

10

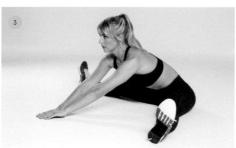

1. Lie on your back with your legs straight out in front of you and your arms by your sides, palms down on the ground.
2. With momentum bring the legs and knees up, rolling back over your head as far as you can comfortably go.
3. From this position spring forwards again, splitting the legs and reaching through the middle with your arms and upper body to create a stretch in your hamstring and adductors. Repeat.

POLE OR WALL SQUAT

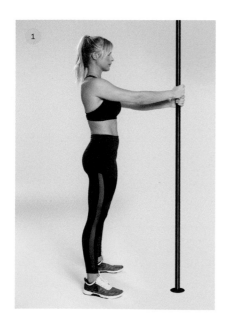

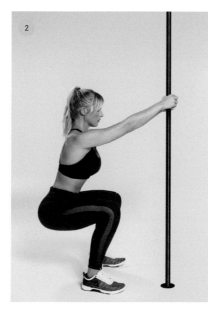

1. Hold on to a pole or wall at arm's length. Have your feet just wider than hip-width apart and slightly turned out.
2. Using the pole to support your body weight, move back into a squat position keeping your upper torso upright. Try to sit deep into the squat without your heels lifting off the floor. Pause for 5 seconds and then slowly come back up to repeat.

 1

 5

YOUR COOL-DOWN STRETCHES

Exercise	Sets	Reps or Time	Target Area
Triceps Stretch	1	15 secs	Triceps
Chest Stretch	1	15 secs	Shoulders
Quad Stretch	1	15 secs	Quads
Hip Flexor Stretch	1	15 secs	Groin
Hamstring Stretch	1	15 secs	Hamstrings
Glute Stretch	1	15 secs	Glutes

 SETS   REPS / TIME

TRICEPS STRETCH

1. Stand upright, lift one arm above your head and bend the elbow to reach down behind your neck towards your upper back with your hand.
2. Use your free hand to gently push the elbow down to increase the stretch. Hold and repeat on the opposite arm.

 1

 15 SECS PER SIDE

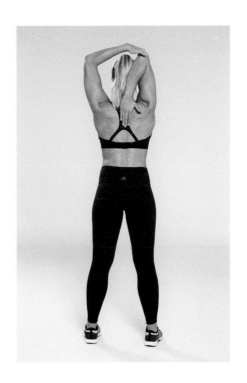

CHEST STRETCH

1. Stand up straight with feet hip-width apart, shoulders square but relaxed. Interlock your fingers behind your back, with your palms facing up, near your glutes.
2. Keeping your back straight push your arms upwards slowly while squeezing your shoulder blades together, holding at your highest point. Repeat.

 1

 15 SECS

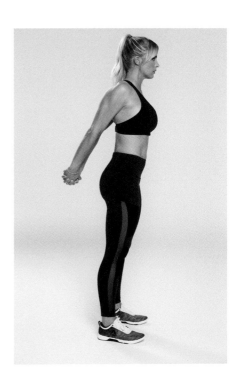

QUAD
STRETCH

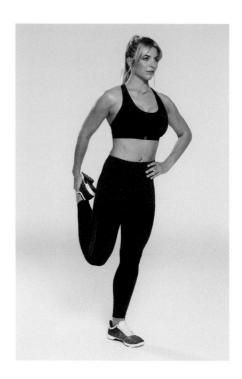

While standing, bend one of your legs behind you, pulling your foot into your bum with one hand. You may need to hold on to a wall for balance. Don't arch the back and keep the pelvis in neutral position. Hold and repeat with the other leg.

 1

 15 SECS PER SIDE

HIP FLEXOR
STRETCH

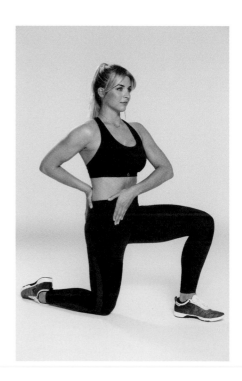

1. From a kneeling position place one foot in front, keeping your back upright (as if you're about to propose to someone!).
2. Lean forward through the hips to feel a stretch in the front of your rear leg. Hold and repeat on the other side.

 1

 15 SECS PER SIDE

HAMSTRING STRETCH

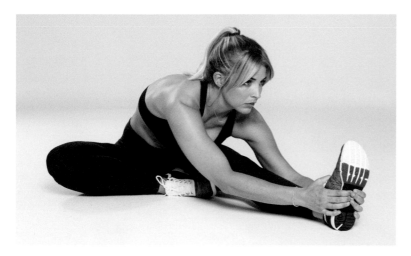

1. From a seated position on the floor place one leg out straight and the other bent, with your foot tucked in towards the top of the straight leg's inside thigh.
2. Lean forwards until you feel a stretch in your hamstrings. Grab the foot furthest away and increase the range if possible. Hold and repeat on the other side.

 1

 15 SECS PER SIDE

GLUTE STRETCH

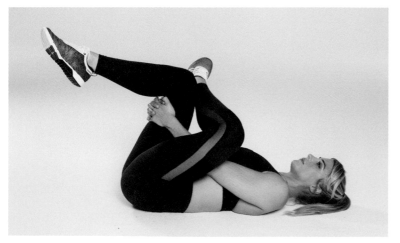

Lie on your back with your knees bent. Lift one ankle up and rest it across the opposite knee. Reach underneath the lower leg and pull it in towards your chest, feeling a stretch on the outer glute of the bent leg. Hold and repeat on the other side.

 1

  15 SECS PER SIDE

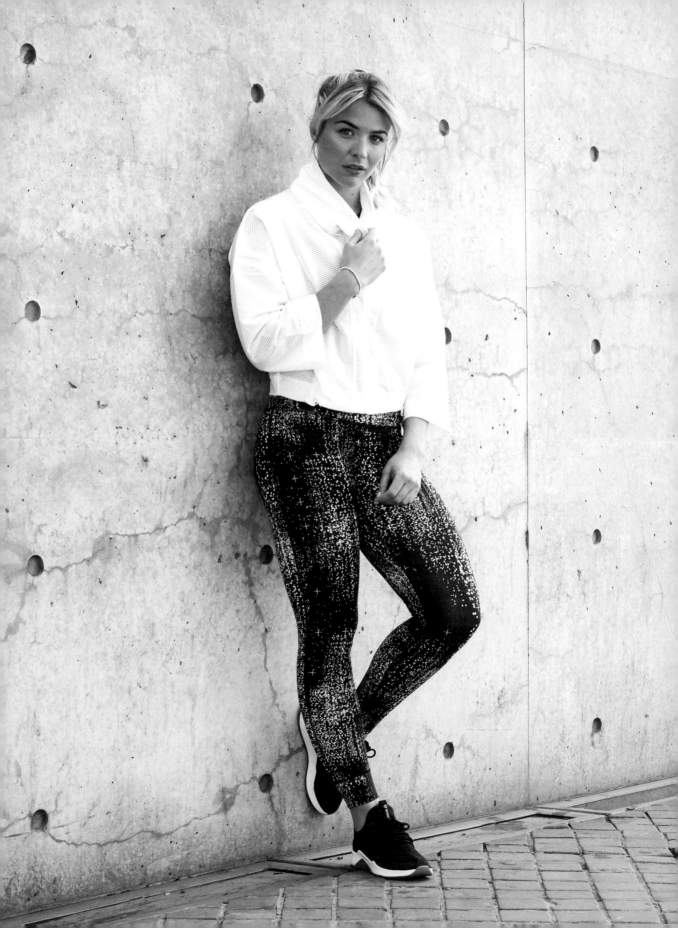

PHASE
ONE

HOME WEIGHTS WORKOUT

WARM UP 5 MINS (PAGE 172)
WORK OUT 35–40 MINS
COOL DOWN 5 MINS (PAGE 176)

Exercise	Sets	Reps or Time	Rest	Target Area
Glute Bridge	3–4	15	40 secs	Glutes & Hamstrings
DB Shoulder Press	3–4	15	40 secs	Shoulders & Triceps
DB Squat to Chair	3–4	15	40 secs	Full Lower Body
DB Bent Over Row	3–4	15	40 secs	Back & Biceps
DB ALT Reverse Lunges	3–4	15	40 secs	Lower Body, mainly Glutes & Hamstrings
Press-ups	3–4	AMRAP	40 secs	Chest & Triceps

 SETS   REPS / TIME   REST

GLUTE BRIDGE

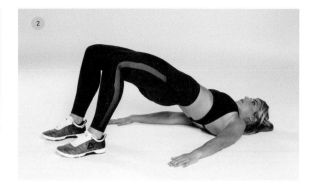

🔄 3–4

⏱ 15 REPS

🏋 40 SECS

1. Begin by lying on your back with knees bent and feet flat on the ground, hip-width apart. Make sure the knees are flexed at a 90-degree angle.
2. Lift your hips up, driving your weight through the heels and squeezing the glutes. Don't arch your lower back. At the top hold for a second,

continuing to squeeze the glutes and making sure your body is in a straight line from knees to shoulders.
3. Slowly lower yourself back down to the starting position, rolling your spine down from the top to bottom as you do. Pause, then repeat.

DB SHOULDER PRESS

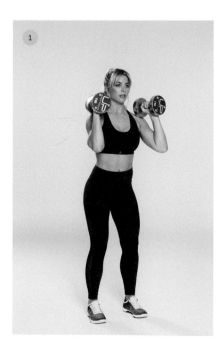
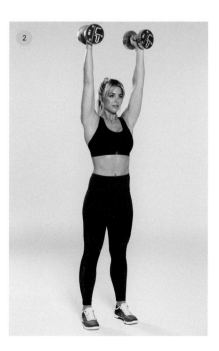

1. Stand with feet shoulder-width apart, holding the dumbbells up at shoulder height with elbows at a 45-degree angle.
2. Drive the dumbbells up to the ceiling, maintaining form by only using your arms, not legs, to drive the weights up (and don't lean back).
3. Pause at the top and slowly return to the starting position and repeat.

🔄 3–4

⏱ 15 REPS

🏋 40 SECS

DB SQUAT TO CHAIR

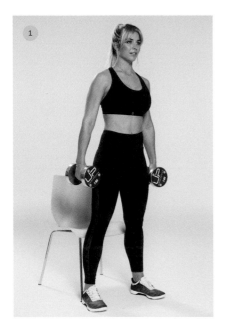

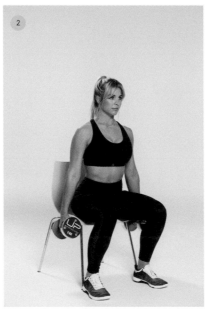

1. Stand in front of a chair with feet shoulder-width apart, back straight, head in a neutral position, holding a set of dumbbells by your side.
2. Bend your knees as if you're going to sit down slowly, moving your hips back onto the chair. Keeping the chest up and back straight go into the seated position.
3. Drive your weight back up through the middle of your feet, without an excessive forward lean, to get back up. At the top squeeze the glutes before repeating.

🔄 3–4

⏱ 15 REPS

🔋 40 SECS

DB BENT OVER ROW

🔄 3–4

⏱ 15 REPS

🔋 40 SECS

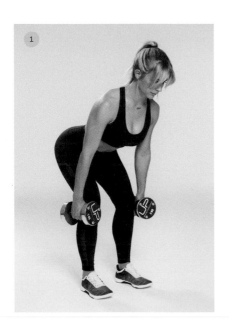

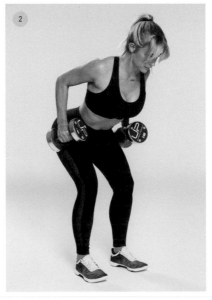

1. Standing and holding a set of dumbbells by your sides, bend your knees slightly and lean forward, lowering your torso towards the ground by bending at the waist. Make sure you keep your back straight and stop when you're pretty much facing the floor. The weights will hang directly in front of you as your arms hang from your shoulder joints.
2. Keeping the head up and torso fixed, lift the elbows up towards the ceiling squeezing the shoulder blades together at the top of the movement.
3. Hold for a second, then slowly lower to the starting position before repeating.

DB ALT REVERSE LUNGES

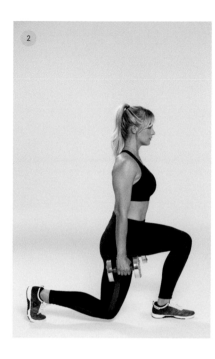

1. Stand with feet shoulder-width apart with your arms by your sides holding a set of dumbbells.
2. Step backwards with one leg, flexing the knee to drop the hips towards the ground. Keep going until your rear knee nearly touches the floor. Keep the spine tall and the weight in your front foot towards the heel.
3. Drive your weight back up through the heel of the front foot and raise yourself back to the starting position to repeat on the other leg.

- 3–4
- 15 REPS
- 40 SECS

PRESS-UPS

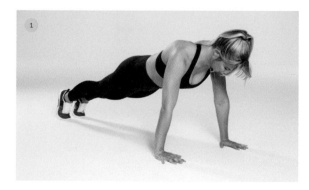

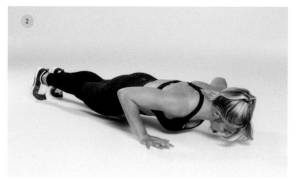

- 3–4
- AMRAP
- 40 SECS

1. Get into a prone position on the floor, supporting your weight through your hands and toes, or alternatively place your kees on the floor.

2. Keeping your back straight, slowly lower yourself until the chest is just about to touch the floor, pushing the elbows away at a 45-degree angle from the side of your torso. Hold this position for a second before driving back to the starting position. Don't round the upper back. You can do these on your knees if full-body is too hard.

HOME HIIT, ABS AND CORE WORKOUT

WARM UP 5 MINS (PAGE 172)
WORK OUT 35–40 MINS
COOL DOWN 5 MINS (PAGE 176)

Exercise	Sets	Reps or Time	Rest	Target Area
Jumping Jacks	5	30 secs	30 secs	Cardiovascular Full Body
Mountain Climbers	5	30 secs	30 secs	Cardiovascular Full Body
High Knees	5	30 secs	30 secs	Cardiovascular Full Body
Lying Leg Raises	3	30 secs	30 secs	Lower Abs
Plank	3	30 secs	30 secs	Core

 SETS REPS / TIME REST

JUMPING JACKS

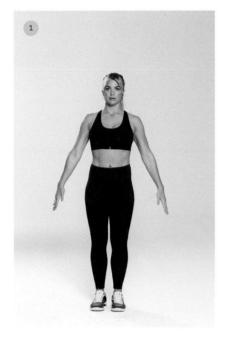

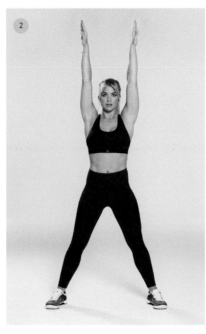

1. Start with feet together and arms by your sides.
2. In one motion jump your feet out laterally and raise your arms above your head, making a star shape.
3. Reverse the motion back to the starting position and repeat.

↻ 5

⏱ 30 SECS

⧗ 30 SECS

MOUNTAIN CLIMBERS

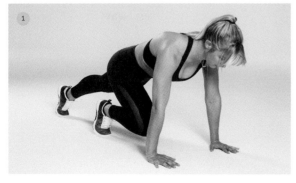

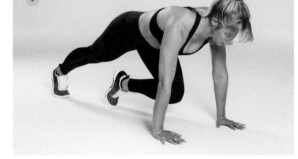

↻ 5

⏱ 30 SECS

⧗ 30 SECS

1. Start in a press-up position with your weight supported by hands and feet. Bring one knee up until it is under the hip to set your starting position.

2. Explosively reverse the position, swapping the legs in a 'climbing' movement. Repeat this movement continuously.

HIGH KNEES

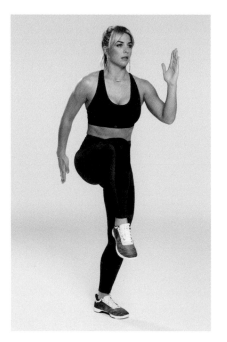
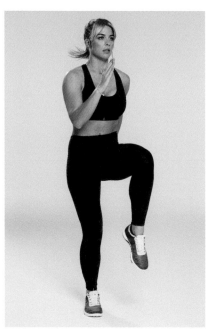

Begin with feet shoulder-width apart and arms bent at your side. Start running on the spot, getting the knees up as high as possible. Stay light and soft on the feet.

↻ 5

⏱ 30 SECS

🕐 30 SECS

LYING LEG RAISES

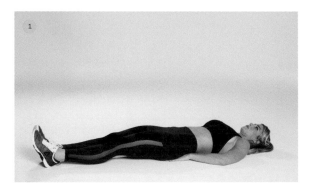
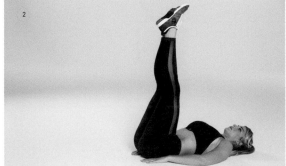

↻ 3

⏱ 30 SECS

🕐 30 SECS

1. Lie with your back on the floor and legs extended out in front of you, with a slight bend in the knee. Place your hands flat on the floor underneath your bum, pushing your weight into them.

2. Raise your legs up together, just past a vertical line position, tucking the pelvis in.
3. Under control, lower the legs back down to the starting position, without letting your heels touch the floor. Repeat. Work to the best range you can, and if you need to, rest your heels down between reps.

PLANK

Get into a prone position on the floor, supporting your weight through your forearms and toes. Make sure the elbows sit directly below the shoulder joints. Lift the hips up so the pelvis is in a neutral position and hold, squeezing the glutes and keeping the abs tight. Hold for the time period set. This is much harder than it sounds! If it's too difficult, repeat on your knees.

↻ 3

⏱ 30 SECS

🕐 30 SECS

'You *can* feel healthier.

You *can* feel stronger.

You *can* feel more confident.'

GYM WEIGHTS WORKOUT

WARM UP 5 MINS (PAGE 172)
WORK OUT 35–40 MINS
COOL DOWN 5 MINS (PAGE 176)

Exercise	Sets	Reps or Time	Rest	Target Area
Barbell Romanian Deadlift (RDL)	3–4	15	40 secs	Glutes & Hamstrings
Dumbbell Seated Shoulder Press	3–4	15	40 secs	Shoulders & Triceps
Walking Barbell Lunges	3–4	15 per leg	40 secs	Full Lower Body
Lat Pull Down	3–4	15	40 secs	Back & Biceps
Leg Curl	3–4	15	40 secs	Hamstrings
Cable Tricep Extension	3–4	15	40 secs	Triceps

 SETS REPS / TIME REST

BARBELL RDL

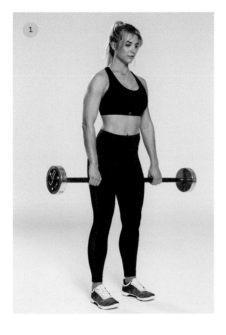

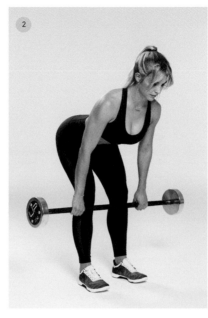

1. Stand up straight with feet shoulder-width apart and hold a barbell in an over-hand position resting against the middle of your upper thighs.
2. Keeping your back straight, hinge the hips, slowly pushing your bum back with only a partial bend in the knees, dropping the barbell slowly towards the floor, under control. You should feel tension in the hamstrings as your hands rotate and approach knee level. Keep your natural spine alignment and don't round the upper back. When the hips can't push back any further, pause, then return to the starting position, and squeeze the glutes hard at the top.

🔄 3–4

⏱ 15 REPS

🏋 40 SECS

DB SEATED SHOULDER PRESS

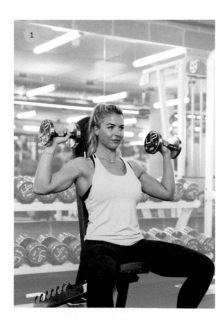

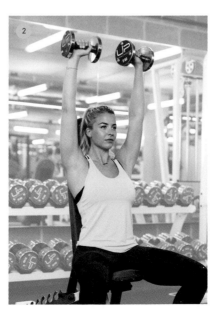

1. Sit on a weight bench that's set at 90 degrees. Hold the dumbbells up at shoulder height with the elbows at a 45-degree angle.
2. Keeping the chest up and shoulder blades back, drive the dumbbells up to the ceiling. Pause at the top and slowly return to the starting position. Repeat.

🔄 3–4

⏱ 15 REPS

🏋 40 SECS

WALKING BARBELL LUNGES

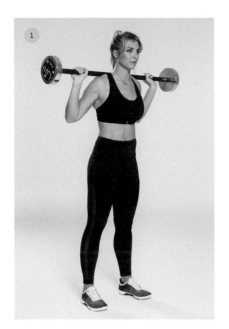
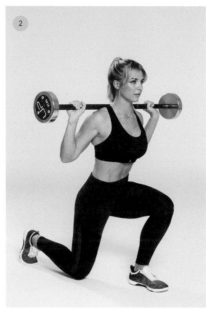

1. Stand with feet shoulder-width apart, holding a small barbell across the top of your shoulders.
2. Step forward with one leg, flexing the knee to drop the hips towards the ground. Keep going until your rear knee nearly touches the ground. Keep the spine tall and track your front knee over its toe line.
3. At this bottom position drive your weight through the heel of the front foot and raise yourself back to the starting position to repeat on the other leg.

 3–4

 15 REPS PER LEG

 40 SECS

LAT PULL DOWN

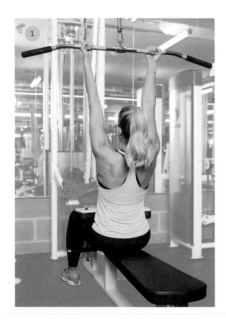
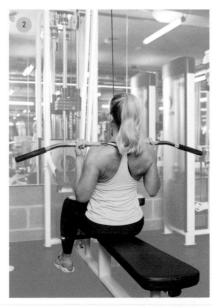

1. Take a shoulder-width underhand grip on the lat pull bar which is attached to the high pulley lat pulldown machine. Lift your chest up towards the ceiling creating a small arch in the lower back.
2. Pull the bar down to the midline of your chest, thinking about driving your elbows down into the ground.
3. Pause and squeeze your shoulder blades together before slowly returning to the starting position under control.

 3–4

 15 REPS

 40 SECS

LEG CURL

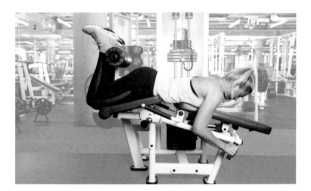

🔄 **3–4**

⏱ **15 REPS**

🔋 **40 SECS**

1. Choose either the lying down leg curl machine or the sitting version. For the lying one: adjust it to suit your height and lie face-down on the bench with the pad of the lever on the back of your legs, just above the Achilles and below the calves. Keeping your torso flat, hold the handles on the side, making sure your legs are fully extended with your feet straight.
2. Curl your legs as far as you can into your glutes without lifting the hips or upper legs from the bench.
3. Hold, then slowly return to the starting position. For a seated machine the same principle applies, just in a seated position!

CABLE TRICEP EXTENSION

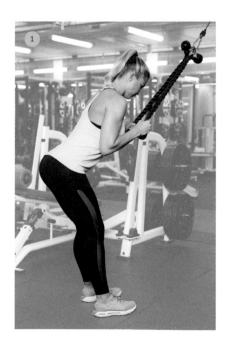 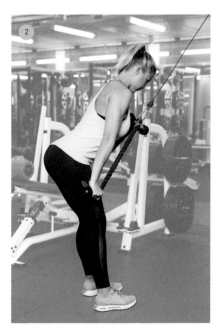

1. Use a rope attachment on the high end of a cable pulley machine. Hold it with a neutral grip (palms facing each other). Stand with the spine straight with a slight forward lean. Keep the upper arms by your side close to the body.
2. Drive your hands down towards your thighs, fully extending the arms and squeezing the triceps at this end range. Don't move the upper arms or allow the elbows to flair out.
3. Pause and slowly return to the starting position to repeat.

🔄 **3–4**

⏱ **15 REPS**

🔋 **40 SECS**

GYM HIIT, ABS AND CORE WORKOUT

WARM UP 5 MINS (PAGE 172)
WORK OUT 35–40 MINS
COOL DOWN 5 MINS (PAGE 176)

Exercise	Sets	Reps or Time	Rest	Target Area
KB Swings	5	30 secs	45 secs	Cardiovascular, mainly Lower Body
Medicine Ball Slams	5	30 secs	45 secs	Cardiovascular Full Body
Swiss Ball Crunch	3–4	15 secs	45 secs	Abs & Core

 SETS   REPS / TIME 🍾 REST

KB SWINGS

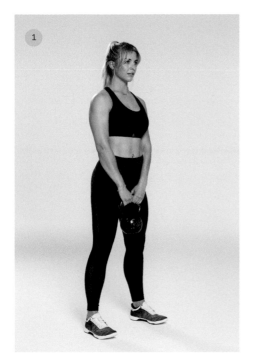

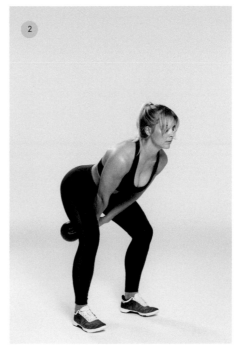

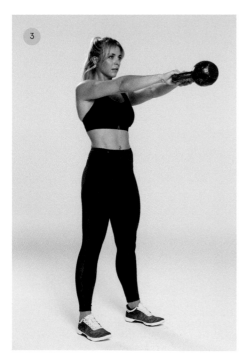

1. Stand with feet shoulder-width apart and hold a kettlebell in the middle of them. Push back with your bum, keeping your back straight and bending the knees slightly to get into position.
2. Holding the kettlebell with both hands, lift it up and swing it back between your legs.
3. Reverse the direction and drive through with the hips, allowing the kettlebell to swing back straight out in front of you as you stand up straight. Don't let your arms go higher than parallel to the floor.
4. At the end range point allow the kettlebell to drop back down in a pendulum style between the legs, crouching down, then repeat the movement. Don't use the shoulders: this is a hip hinge movement. You need to use a fairly hefty kettlebell weight for this exercise to challenge yourself. Although this exercise utilises weights it's actually traditionally more of a cardio exercise so works best in this section.

 5

 30 SECS

 45 SECS

MEDICINE BALL SLAMS

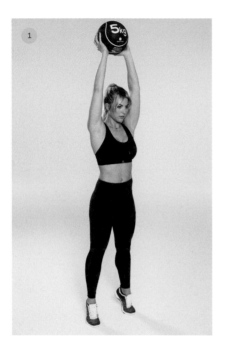
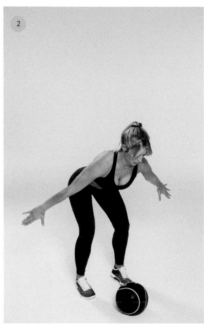

1. Stand with feet set shoulder-width apart, holding a medicine ball with both hands at waist-height. Start the move by raising the ball up above your head, fully extending the body.
2. Slam the ball down into the ground in front of you as hard as possible. Retrieve the ball and repeat the movement.

5

30 SECS

45 SECS

SWISS BALL CRUNCH

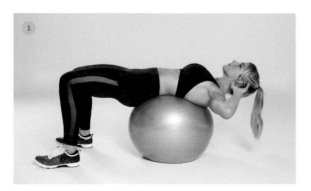
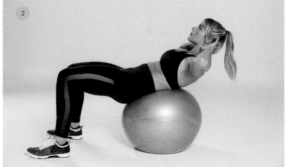

3–4

15 SECS

45 SECS

1. Lie over a Swiss ball with your lower back curvature pressed against the round surface of the ball. Your legs should be bent at the knee with your feet firmly pressed against the floor for stability. Your upper body should be hanging just over the top of the ball. Place your hands either by your temples or across your chest. Lower your upper body over the ball to stretch the abs – this is your starting position for all reps.
2. Keeping the hips still, crunch the upper body upwards by flexing at the waist and contracting the abs. The lower back must always remain in contact with the ball. Breathe out as you come up and then in on the way back down to the starting position. To increase intensity, you can hold a weight plate across your chest.

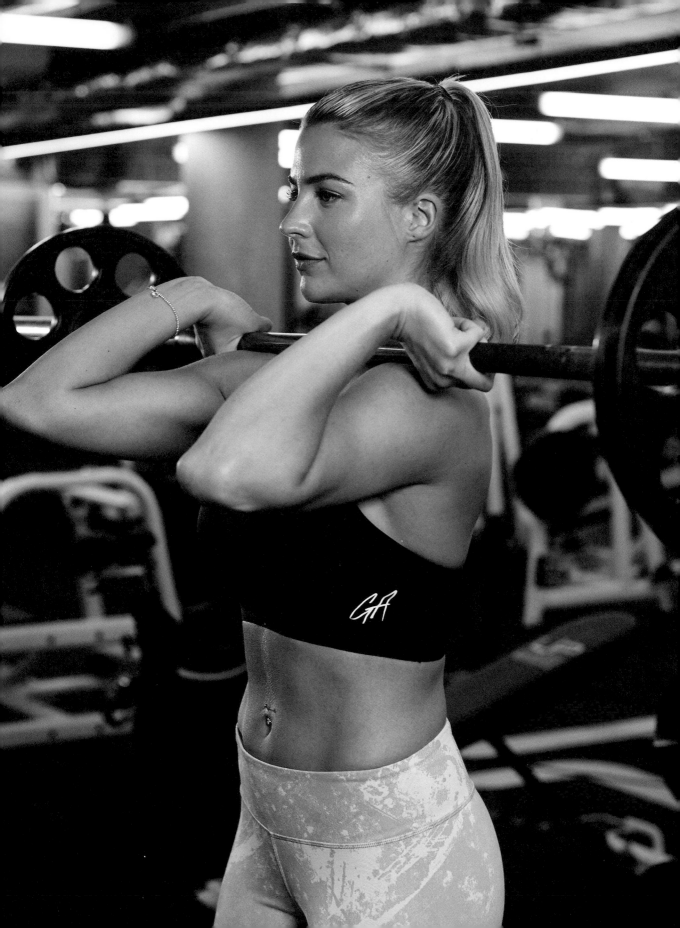

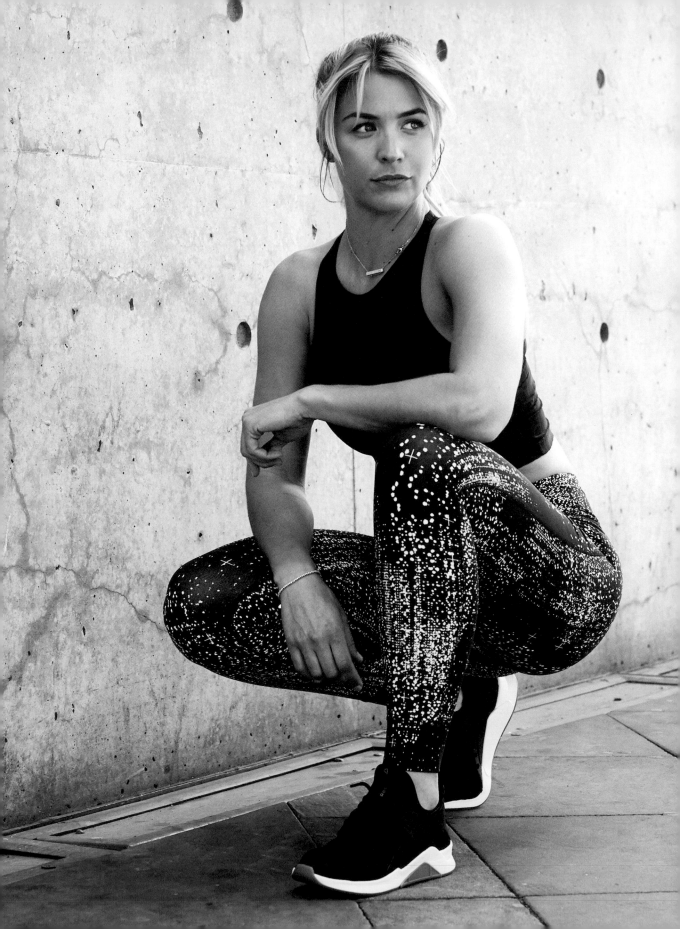

PHASE
TWO

PHASE TWO TRAINING PLAN

HOME WEIGHTS WORKOUT

WARM UP 5 MINS (PAGE 172)
WORK OUT 35–40 MINS
COOL DOWN 5 MINS (PAGE 176)

Exercise	Sets	Reps or Time	Rest	Target Area
Single Leg Glute Bridge	3–4	15 per leg	40 secs	Glutes & Hamstrings
Single Leg Dumbbell RDL	3–4	15 per leg	40 secs	Glutes & Hamstrings
Dumbbell Bent Over Row	3–4	15	40 secs	Upper Back & Biceps
Dumbbell Side Lateral Raises	3–4	15	40 secs	Shoulders
Dumbbell Forward Lunges	3–4	15 per leg	40 secs	Lower Body, mainly Quads
Floor Dumbbell Tricep Ext	3–4	15	40 secs	Triceps

 SETS   REPS / TIME   REST

SINGLE LEG GLUTE BRIDGE

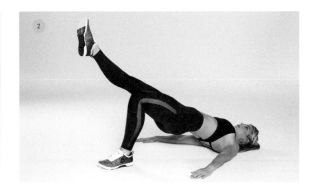

🔄 3–4

⏱ 15 REPS
PER LEG

🔋 40 SECS

1. This exercise is a progression from the Glute Bridge exercise in Phase 1 (page 183). Lie on your back on the ground. Place both feet on the floor with knees bent.
2. Elevate one leg in the air so it is almost straight. With the other leg drive your hips up into the air pushing your weight down and through the heel of the fixed leg. Taking the hips as far as you can without arching the lower back, squeeze the working glute as hard as you can.
3. Control the lowering phase back to the starting position and repeat for the desired number of reps, then repeat with the other leg.

SINGLE LEG DB RDL

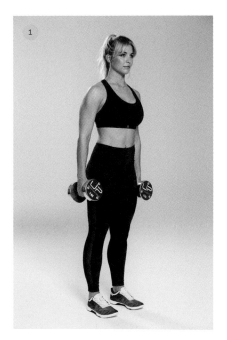

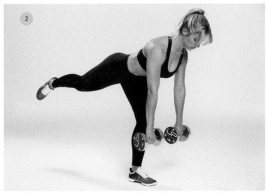

🔄 3–4

⏱ 15 REPS
PER LEG

🔋 40 SECS

1. Stand with feet hip-width apart, with knees slightly bent, holding a set of dumbbells by your sides. Lift one leg off the floor and maintain balance.
2. Flexing at the hips, start to lean forwards while simultaneously taking the lifted leg backwards as a counterbalance, keeping it relatively straight, arms swinging naturally towards the floor. Keep moving until your torso is parallel with floor, making sure you don't arch the lower back – you should feel a stretch in the hamstring.
3. Pause at the end position before returning to the starting position and repeating with the other leg. You can touch down with your non-working leg between reps to maintain balance.

DB BENT OVER ROW

3–4

3–4

15 REPS

40 SECS

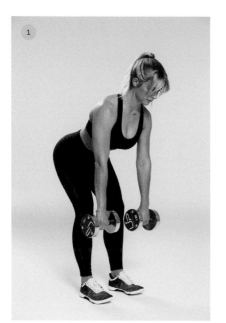

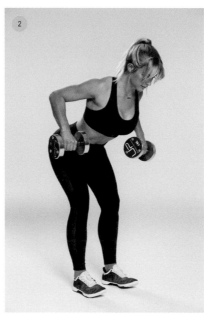

1. The semi-pronated grip targets the upper back as opposed to the mid-back from Phase 1 (see page 184). Standing and holding a set of dumbbells by your sides, bend your knees slightly and lower your torso down towards the ground by pushing the hips back, bending at the waist. Make sure you keep your back straight and take it down until it's almost parallel with the floor. The weight will hang directly in front of you as your arms hang from your shoulder joints. Turn your hands so they are at a 45-degree angle from your torso.
2. Keeping the head up and torso fixed, lift the elbows up towards the ceiling, squeezing the shoulder blades at the top of the movement. The elbows should be at a 45-degree angle from the body as you perform this lift.
3. Hold for a second, then slowly lower to the starting position before repeating.

DB SIDE LATERAL RAISES

3–4

15 REPS

40 SECS

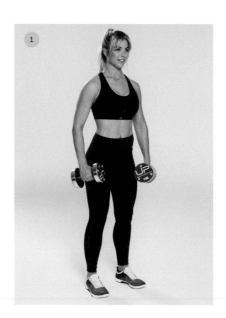

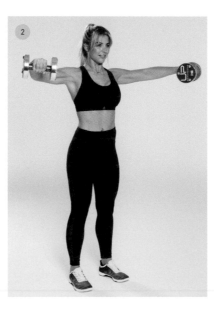

1. Standing with feet hip-width apart, chest up, shoulder blades back, hold a set of dumbbells by your sides in a neutral grip, palms facing each other.
2. Without swinging, lift the dumbbells to your sides, away from your body, with a slight bend in the elbows and the hands tilting forward as if you were pouring water from a jug into a glass. Keep lifting until your arms are parallel to the floor, at shoulder height, without arching your lower back.
3. Pause at this top end position and then, under control, lower the weights back to the starting position. Repeat.

DB FORWARD LUNGES

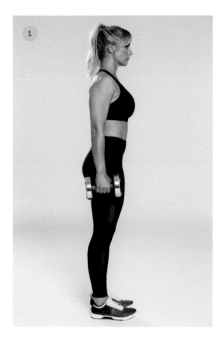
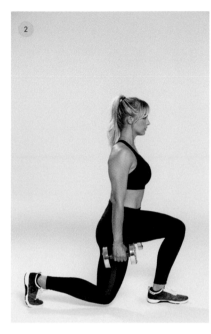

1. Stand upright with feet hip-width apart and your hands by your sides holding a set of dumbbells. Keep your chest up and shoulder blades back and take a moderate-length step forward with one foot.
2. Under control, lower yourself towards the floor until your back knee is about to touch the ground. Your front knee should be at a 90-degree angle and tracking over the front foot toe line.
3. Pause and then drive your weight through the front foot pushing yourself backwards to the starting position. You can either alternate lunges or work one leg before the other.

- 3–4
- 15 REPS PER LEG
- 40 SECS

FLOOR DB TRICEP EXT

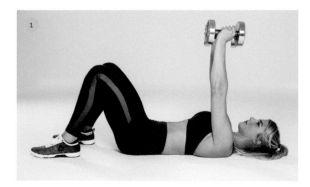
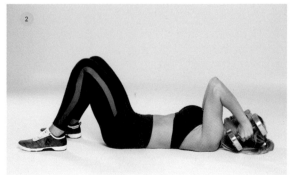

- 3–4
- 15 REPS
- 40 SECS

1. Lie on the floor with your back on the ground and the legs bent at the knees. Hold a set of dumbbells directly above the shoulder joints in a neutral position with the palms facing each other.
2. From this starting position slowly lower the dumbbells down towards the front part of the shoulders without allowing the upper arms to move forwards or backwards or rotate. Stop just short of touching the shoulders.
3. Use the triceps to drive the weight back up to the starting position locking the arms and squeezing the triceps at the top end. Pause and repeat, avoiding your head at all times.

HOME HIIT, ABS & CORE WORKOUT

WARM UP 5 MINS (PAGE 172)
WORK OUT 35–40 MINS
COOL DOWN 5 MINS (PAGE 176)

Exercise	Sets	Reps or Time	Rest	Target Area
Jumping Alternating Lunges	5	30 secs	30 secs	Cardiovascular Lower Body
Double Leg Lateral Bounds	5	30 secs	30 secs	Cardiovascular Lower Body
Burpees	5	30 secs	30 secs	Cardiovascular Full Body
Side Plank with Top Leg Elevation	4	5–10 per side	30 secs	Core / Obliques / Hip Abductors
Flutter Kicks	4	30 secs	30 secs	Abs & Core

 SETS   REPS / TIME   REST

JUMPING ALT LUNGES

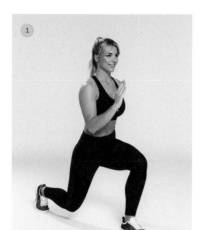
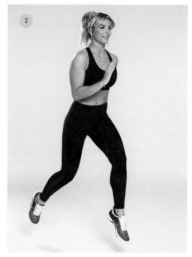
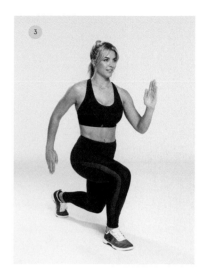

🔄 5

⏱ 30 SECS

🕐 30 SECS

1. Set up in a lunge stance position with one foot forwards and the knee bent with the rear knee almost touching the ground.
2. Extending through both legs, jump up as high as possible, swinging your arms to gain extra lift. Once clear of the floor switch the position of your legs, moving the lead leg back and rear leg forward.
3. Make a controlled soft landing (landing toes first, rather than on your heels) absorbing the impact back into a lunge position. Repeat.

DOUBLE LEG LATERAL BOUNDS

🔄 5

⏱ 30 SECS

🕐 30 SECS

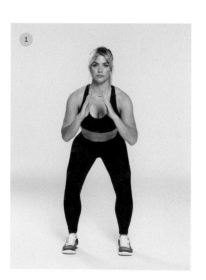
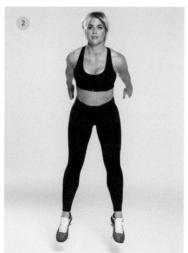
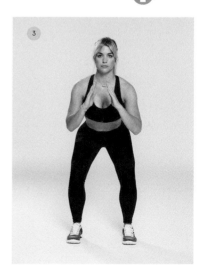

1. Get into a half squat position, facing forward.
2. Jump sideways off your outward facing leg as far as possible before landing on both feet.
3. Immediately repeat on the other leg so you are 'bounding' from one side to the other.

BURPEES

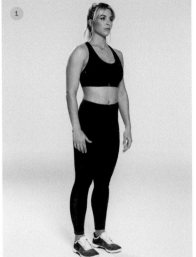 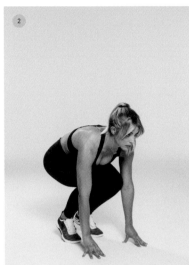

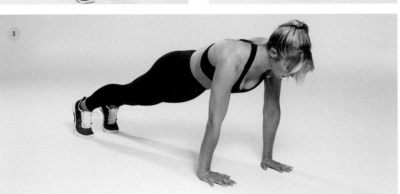

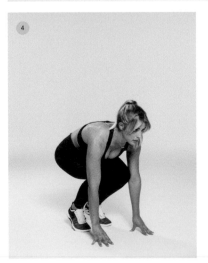

1. Stand with feet shoulder-width apart.
2. Drop your hands down to the floor, taking your weight.
3. Quickly kick your feet out into a press-up position.
4. Jump your feet back under the hips.
5. Explode back into a standing position, jumping into the air and raising your hands. Repeat.

 3–4

 30 SECS

 30 SECS

SIDE PLANK WITH TOP LEG ELEVATION

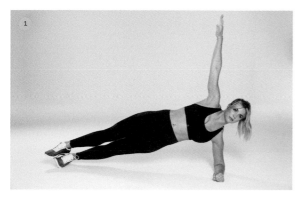

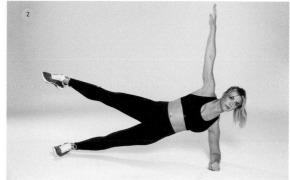

○ 4

⏱ 5–10 REPS PER SIDE

◑ 30 SECS

1. Lie on your side with your weight resting on your elbow, hips and feet. Keep the back straight and your head in a neutral position. From here, lift your hips towards the ceiling to create a straight line from head to toe down the centre of your body.

2. Brace the core and squeeze the glutes and then lift your top leg away from the other leg as high as possible for the set number of reps. If this is too difficult you can start as above but with the knees on the floor and the legs bent at a 90-degree angle.

FLUTTER KICKS

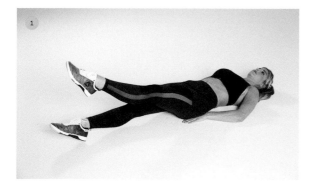

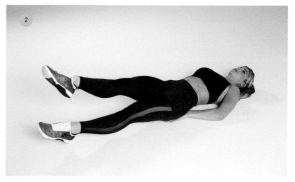

○ 4

⏱ 30 SECS

◑ 30 SECS

1. Lie on your back with your legs straight and place your hands under your glutes, palms facing down.

2. Raise both legs off the floor about 38–50cm (15–20in) and contract your abs. From here, kick your legs up and down as if you were swimming.

GYM WEIGHTS WORKOUT

In Phase 2, readers should now be lifting slightly heavier weights, which is why the number of sets and reps have decreased.

WARM UP 5 MINS (PAGE 172)
WORK OUT 35–40 MINS
COOL DOWN 5 MINS (PAGE 176)

Exercise	Sets	Reps or Time	Rest	Target Area
Barbell Rack Pulls	3–4	10	40 secs	Glutes, Hamstrings & Lower Back
Dumbbell Incline Chest Press	3–4	10	40 secs	Chest, Shoulders & Triceps
Dumbbell Split Squats	3–4	10 per leg	40 secs	Glutes, Hamstrings & Quads
Single Arm Dumbbell Row	3–4	10 per arm	40 secs	Back & Biceps
Barbell Glute Bridge	3–4	10	40 secs	Glutes
Incline Dumbbell Tricep Extension	3–4	10	40 secs	Triceps

 SETS REPS / TIME 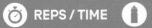 REST

BARBELL RACK PULLS

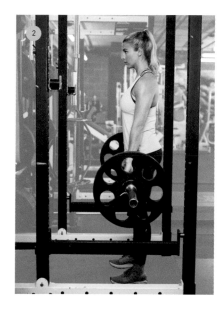

⟳ 3–4

⏱ 10 REPS

🕐 40 SECS

1. Set up in a squat rack with a bar set on the pins just below knee height. With a shoulder-width grip and feet hip-width apart, set the hips back and position yourself as shown.
2. Keeping the head forward, brace your core and extend through the hips and knees pulling the bar up. At the top squeeze the glutes, drop the chin and keep the shoulder blades back. Don't arch the lower back or lean back at the top position.
3. Control the down movement and repeat.

DB INCLINE CHEST PRESS

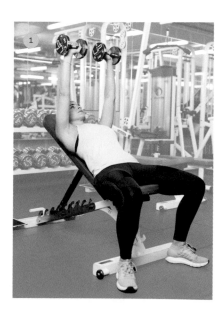

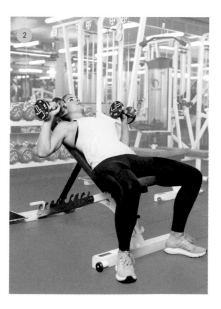

⟳ 3–4

⏱ 10 REPS

🕐 40 SECS

1. Set a bench to an incline of 45 degrees. Lie back on the bench with a set of dumbbells in each hand. Lift the weights so they are directly above the shoulder joints. Squeeze your shoulder blades together and create a small arch in your lower back.
2. Slowly lower the weights down towards the chest, stopping when you can feel a good stretch, pause, then drive the weight back up to the top position. Don't round or flatten the upper back. Pause, then repeat.

DB SPLIT SQUATS

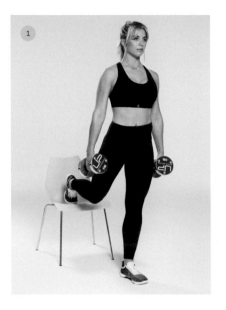
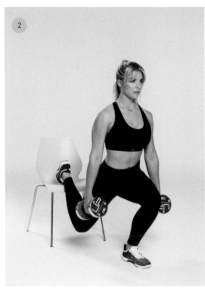

🔄 3–4

⏱ 10 REPS PER LEG

🔋 40 SECS

1. Stand with one foot flat on the floor and with the back foot on a chair so the heel is slightly elevated. Keep the chest up and shoulder blades back; your hips and shoulders should remain parallel, facing forwards.
2. Slowly lower your back knee towards the ground until you reach 90 degrees, stopping just before you touch the ground.
3. Pause, then drive back up through the front leg to the starting position. Repeat for the desired number of reps for both legs.

SINGLE ARM DB ROW

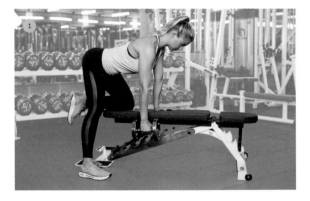
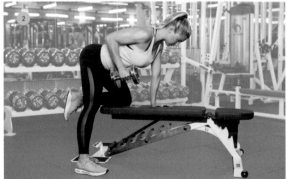

🔄 3–4

⏱ 10 REPS PER ARM

🔋 40 SECS

1. Use a flat bench and place one leg on the top end, bending your torso from the waist until your upper body is parallel with the floor. Use the arm of the same side of your leg to hold the other end of the bench for support. Hold the dumbbell in the opposite arm in a neutral grip, keeping your back flat.

2. Pull the weight up in a straight line. Keep the elbow close to the body and think about driving the weight up towards the ceiling using the back not the arm. The torso must remain stationary. Pause at the top without flexing the wrists, then lower the weight back down under control to repeat.

BARBELL GLUTE BRIDGE

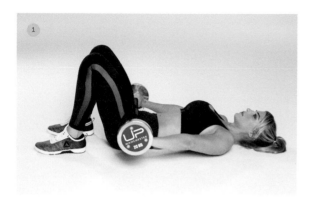

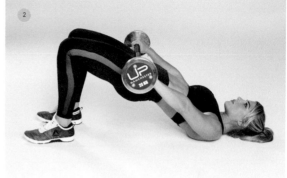

⟳ 3–4

⏱ 10 REPS

🏋 40 SECS

1. Start in a seated position on the floor with a loaded barbell across the legs. You may wish to use a pad on the bar for support. Roll the bar up so it sits directly above the hips and lower yourself flat on the ground. Bring the feet up towards your bum.

2. Drive the hips up towards the ceiling as far as possible by pushing your weight through the heels and keeping your upper back on the ground. Squeeze the glutes at the top without arching the lower back and slowly guide the weight back down to the ground to repeat.

INCLINE DB TRICEP EXTENSION

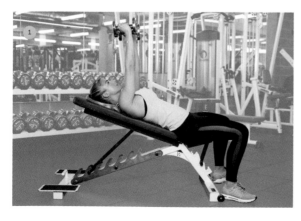

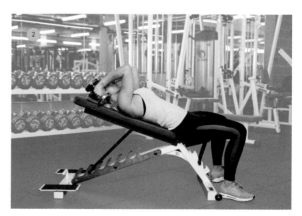

⟳ 3–4

⏱ 10 REPS

🏋 40 SECS

1. Lie on an incline weight bench set at a 45-degree angle. Hold the dumbbells directly above the shoulder joints in a neutral position with palms facing each other.

2. Slowly lower the dumbbells down towards the front part of the shoulders without allowing the upper arms to move forwards or backwards or rotate. Stop just short of touching the shoulders, then use the triceps to drive the weight back up to the starting position, locking the arms and squeezing the triceps at the top end. Pause and repeat, avoiding your head at all times.

GYM HIIT, ABS & CORE WORKOUT

The LISS here is used as a warm-up for the following HIIT workout. You can't go straight into this type of HIIT without doing a slower movement pattern of the exercise beforehand. Likewise, it serves well as the cool-down, burning a good amount of calories collectively. Please disregard the usual warm-up and cool-down workouts you've been asked to do during this section.

Exercise	Sets	Reps or Time	Rest	Target Area
LISS – Hill Walk or Rower	1	5 min	-	Cardiovascular Fitness
HIIT – Treadmill Sprints or Rower Sprints	10	20 secs	40 secs	Anaerobic Fitness
LISS – Hill Walk or Rower	1	5 min	30 secs	Cardiovascular Fitness
Swiss Ball Knee Tucks	3–4	5–10	30 secs	Abs & Core
Decline Ab Crunch – weighted if needed	3–4	5–10	30 secs	Abs

 SETS   REPS / TIME   🚰 REST

LISS – HILL WALK OR ROWER

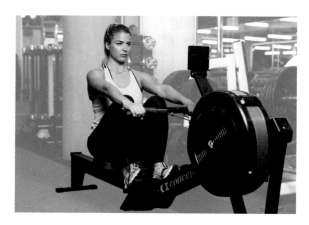

Using either the rower or the treadmill, work at 50–60% of your max HR, working just hard enough to sweat slightly. This is your warm-up for the HIIT ahead.

  1

🕐 5 MINS

HIIT – TREADMILL SPRINTS OR ROWER SPRINTS

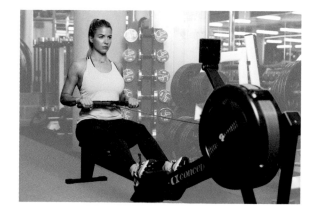

For the rower, keep good posture – back straight, chest upright – and go as fast as possible for the set period of time. You can either rest or row slowly as part of your recovery between rounds. HIIT must be performed with maximum intensity, no holding back. If you're using a treadmill do either sprints or dead treads. If you opt for sprints, keep the belt running and jump your feet to the side to rest, so you don't lose time increasing and decreasing speed. For dead treads you power the belt yourself, solely by running, without turning it on.

 10

 20 SECS

 40 SECS

SWISS BALL KNEE TUCKS

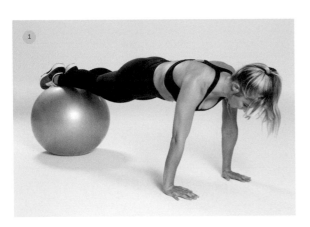

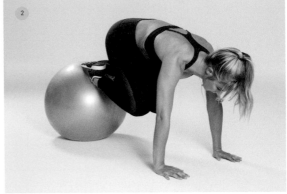

⟳ 3–4

⏱ 5–10 REPS

🗍 30 SECS

1. Kneeling behind a Swiss ball, roll yourself over the ball so you are in a press-up position, hands shoulder-width apart with the ball resting on your shins. Have your legs about hip-width part.

2. Pull your knees into your chest as far as you can by contracting your abs. Hold, then return to the starting position to repeat.

DECLINE AB CRUNCH

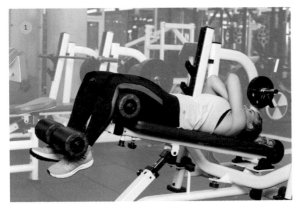

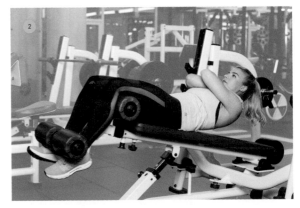

⟳ 3–4

⏱ 5–10 REPS

🗍 30 SECS

1. Lie with your back flat against the pad of the bench with your feet at the highest point, and head at the lowest. Place your hands either by your temples or across your chest.

2. While pushing your lower back down into the bench, begin to roll and lift your shoulders. Breathing out on the way up, contract the abs as hard as you can, rising 10–12cm (4–5in) from the bench with your upper body only. Your lower back should always keep contact with the pad.

3. Pause, then slowly lower yourself back to the starting position. To increase difficulty simply hold a weight plate across your chest.

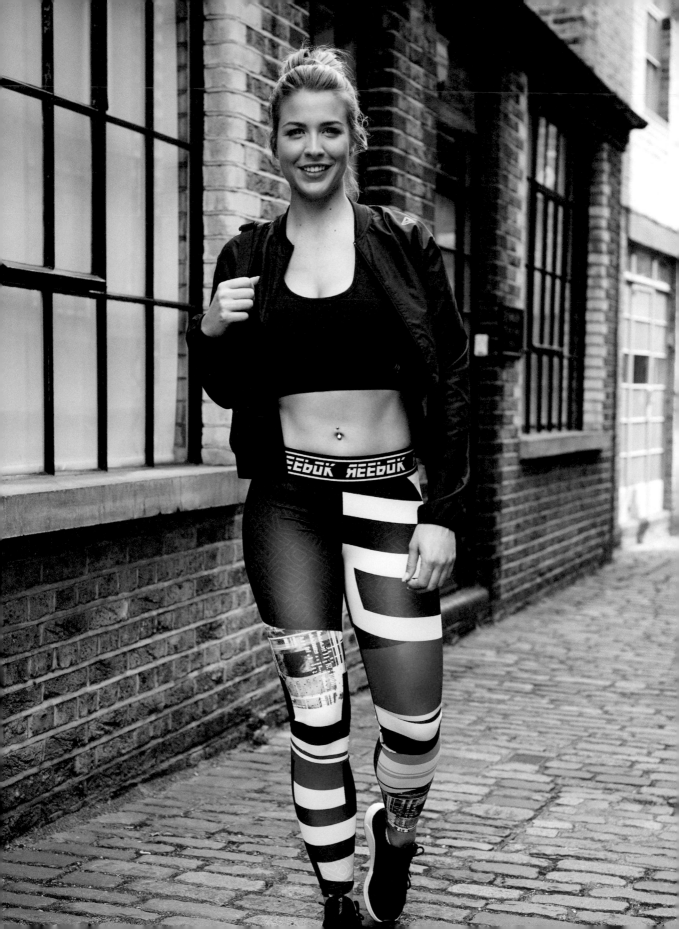

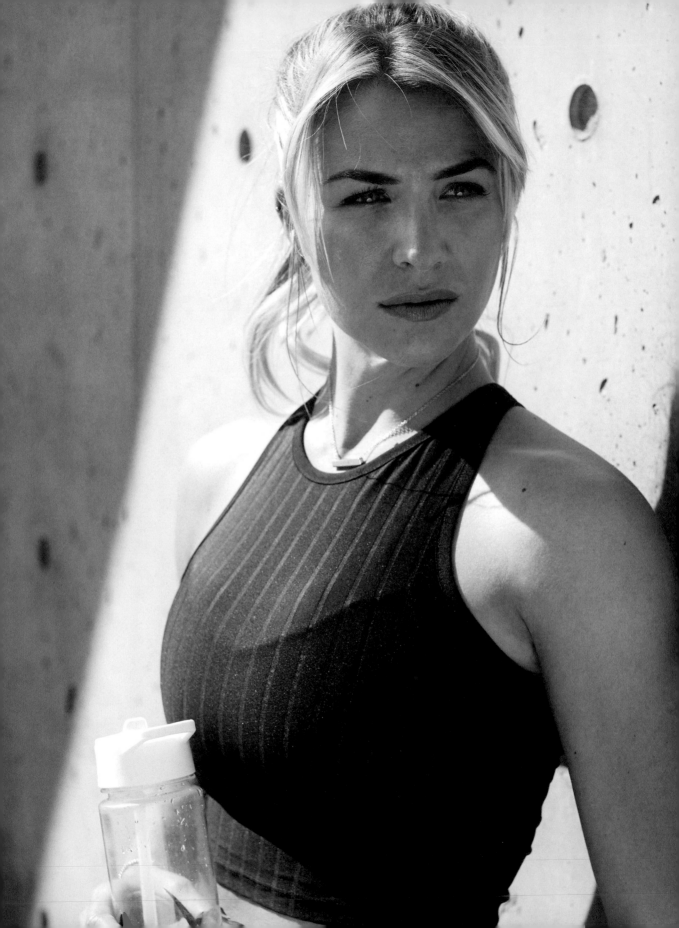

PHASE
THREE

HOME WEIGHTS WORKOUT

WARM UP 5 MINS (PAGE 172)
WORK OUT 35–40 MINS
COOL DOWN 5 MINS (PAGE 176)

Exercise	Sets	Reps or Time	Rest	Target Area
Dumbbell Stiff Leg Deadlift	3–4	15	30 secs	Glutes & Hamstrings
Straight Arm Floor DB Pull Over	3–4	10–15	30 secs	Lats & Chest
Dumbbell Front Squat into Dumbbell Push Press	3–4	10–15	45 secs	Shoulders & Full Lower Body
Dumbbell Side Lunge	3–4	10–15 per leg	30 secs	Lower Body including Adductors
Press-ups	3–4	10–15	30 secs	Triceps & Chest

 SETS REPS / TIME REST

DB STIFF LEG DEADLIFT

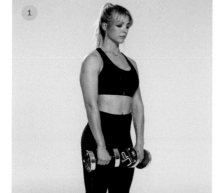

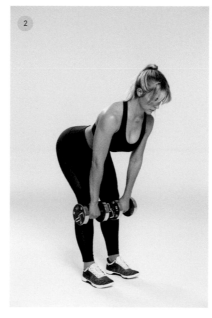

⟳ 3–4

⏱ 15 REPS

⏲ 30 SECS

1. Stand up straight with feet hip-width apart and hold a set of dumbbells with a slight bend in the knees.
2. Keeping the knees fixed, slowly lower the dumbbells towards your feet by hinging the hips away from you, keeping the back straight. Keep moving forwards towards the ground until you feel a stretch in the hamstrings.
3. Pause at your end range without arching or rounding the back and then start to bring yourself back up to the starting position, squeezing the glutes at the top. Pause and repeat. This is similar to the RDL, but with more focus on the hamstring insertion into the glutes.

STRAIGHT ARM FLOOR DB PULL OVER

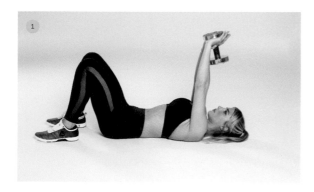

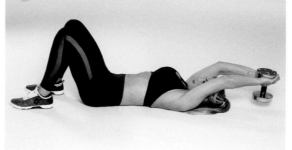

⟳ 3–4

⏱ 10–15 REPS

⏲ 30 SECS

1. Lie on your back with legs bent and feet flat on the floor. Hold one dumbbell with both hands at arm's length over the top of your chest.

2. Keeping the arms straight, slowly lower the dumbbell backwards over your head towards the ground. Take it as far as you can without touching the floor, pause for a second and then, under control, bring it back to the starting position. Keep the arms straight.

DB FRONT SQUAT INTO DB PUSH PRESS

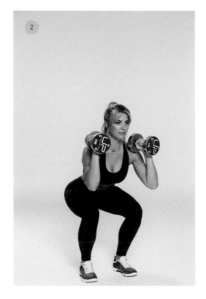

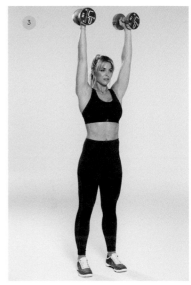

3–4

10–15 REPS

45 SECS

1. Stand with feet shoulder-width apart, holding a set of dumbbells on the top of your shoulders with palms facing each other.
2. Keeping your back straight and chest and head up, squat down towards the ground.

3. At the point your thighs are parallel with the floor, pause and drive the hips back to the starting position while simultaneously pressing the dumbbells straight up towards the ceiling. Don't rotate the palms. Allow the dumbbells to return to your starting position before repeating the movement.

'Do this to feel happier, healthier and more confident within yourself.'

DB SIDE LUNGE

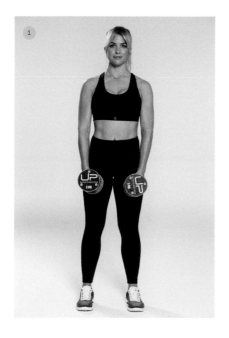

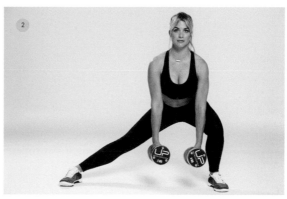

 3–4

 10–15 PER LEG

30 SECS

1. Stand upright with feet shoulder-width apart, holding a set of dumbbells by your sides, palms facing each other. Keep your shoulders back and chest up with a slight bend in the knees.
2. Take a big step out to your side turning your foot out just a little; making sure you stay facing forwards and as upright as possible. Bend the front foot, lowering yourself into a squat while keeping your trailing leg straight.
3. Push back up to the starting position with the bent leg and repeat on the other side.

PRESS-UPS

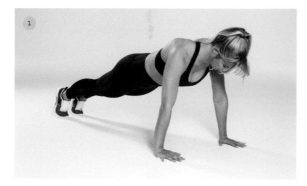

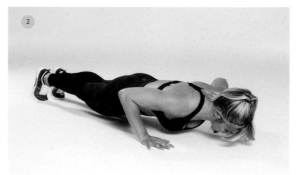

1. Get into a prone position on the floor, supporting your weight through your hands and toes, or alternatively place your knees on the floor.
2. Keeping your back straight, slowly lower yourself until the chest is just about to touch the floor, pushing the elbows away at a 45-degree angle from the side of your torso. Hold this position for a second before driving back to the starting position. Don't round the upper back. This is a great chance to see how much you've improved since Phase One!

 3–4

 AMPRAP

40 SECS

HOME HIIT, ABS & CORE WORKOUT

WARM UP 5 MINS (PAGE 172)
WORK OUT 35–40 MINS
COOL DOWN 5 MINS (PAGE 176)

Exercise	Sets	Reps or Time	Rest	Target Area
Mountain Climbers with Twist	5	30 secs	30 secs	Cardiovascular Full Body
Ice Skaters	5	30 secs	30 secs	Cardiovascular Lower Body
Burpees with Tuck Jump	5	30 secs	30 secs	Cardiovascular Full Body
Plank Step Ups	3	30 secs	30 secs	Core & Upper Body
Jackknife Crunches	3	30 secs	30 secs	Abs & Core

 SETS   REPS / TIME   REST

MOUNTAIN CLIMBERS WITH TWIST

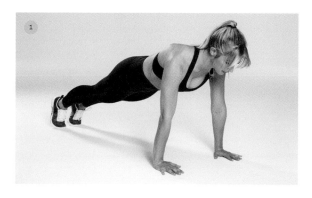
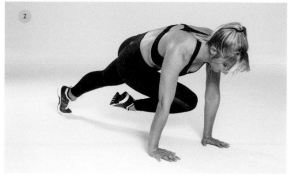

⟳ 5

⏱ 30 SECS

◉ 30 SECS

1. Start in a press-up position with your weight supported by your hands and feet.

2. Flexing the knee and the hip, bring the right knee up towards your left elbow. From here explosively reverse the position of your legs, bringing the left to the right elbow. Repeat this movement continuously for the set time.

ICE SKATERS

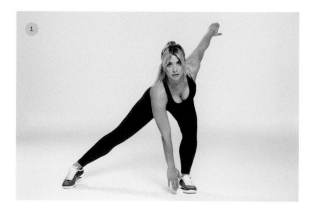
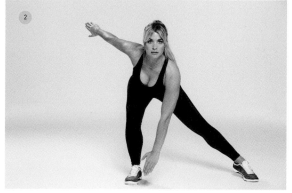

⟳ 5

⏱ 30 SECS

◉ 30 SECS

1. Get into a half squat position facing 90 degrees from your direction of travel. Begin the exercise by jumping to the right with a slight bend in your knees. In the same motion reach down towards the inside of your right foot with your left hand.

2. Load and jump across to the other side to repeat with the opposite hand. Stay light on the feet with a smooth controlled flow to the movement.

BURPEES WITH TUCK JUMP

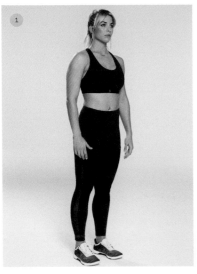

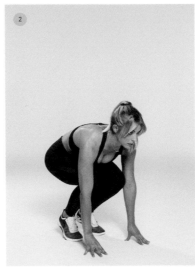

1. Stand with feet shoulder-width apart.
2. Drop your hands down to the floor, taking your weight.
3. Quickly kick your feet out into a press-up position.
4. Jump your feet back under the hips.
5. Perform a small squat to load your weight into the ground. From here jump up into the air as high as you can, bringing your knees up and using your arms to gain power. Ensure a good soft landing by bending the knees slightly upon impact before repeating the process.

 5

 30 SECS

 30 SECS

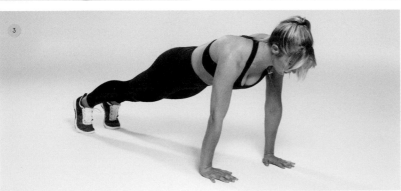

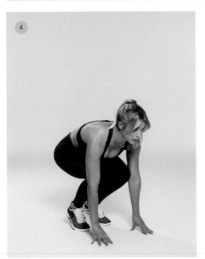

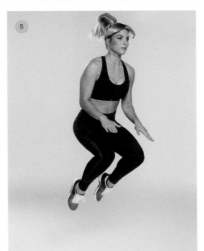

PLANK STEP UPS

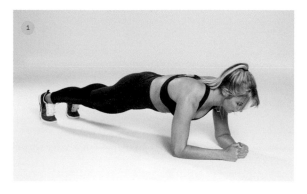

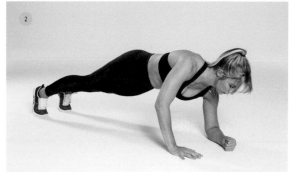

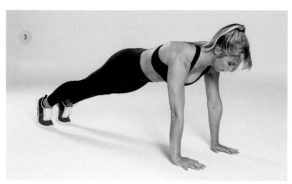

🔄 **3**

⏱️ **30 SECS**

🔋 **30 SECS**

1. Get into a prone position on the floor, supporting your weight through your forearms and toes. Make sure the elbows sit directly below the shoulder joints. Lift up your hips so the pelvis is in a neutral position and hold, squeezing the glutes and keeping the abs tight.
2. Press your body up into a press-up position one arm at a time.
3. Once in the press-up position move back down to the plank position and continue to do this for the set amount of time.

JACKKNIFE CRUNCHES

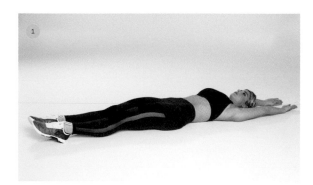

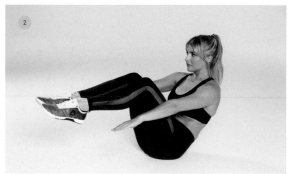

🔄 **3**

⏱️ **30 SECS**

🔋 **30 SECS**

1. Lie flat on your back on the ground with your arms fully extended behind your head and legs out straight.
2. Bend your legs up towards your stomach, stopping when they're at 90 degrees,

whilst bringing your arms towards them, keeping them straight. Straighten your legs and reach your fingers towards your toes so your upper body raises off the floor.
3. With your core engaged and a straight back, lower yourself slowly back to the starting position.

GYM WEIGHTS WORKOUT

WARM UP 5 MINS (PAGE 172)
WORK OUT 35–40 MINS
COOL DOWN 5 MINS (PAGE 176)

Exercise	Sets	Reps or Time	Rest	Target Area
Kettlebell Single Leg RDL	3–4	10 per leg	40 secs	Glutes & Hamstrings
Kettlebell Single Arm Shoulder Press	3–4	10 per arm	40 secs	Shoulders & Triceps
Wide Stance Leg Press	3–4	10	40 secs	Full Lower Body
Cable Face Pulls	3–4	10	40 secs	Upper Back
Dumbbell Step Ups	3–4	15 per leg	40 secs	Glutes, Hamstrings & Quads
Overhead Cable Tricep Extension	3–4	15	40 secs	Triceps

 SETS REPS / TIME ⬤ REST

KB SINGLE LEG RDL

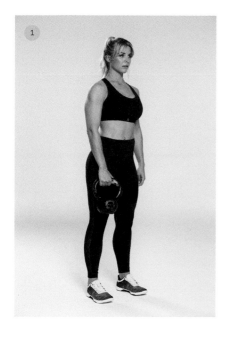

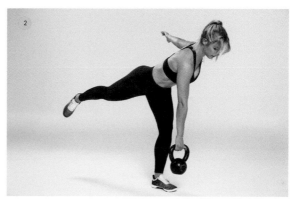

3–4

10 PER LEG

40 SECS

1. Start by standing and holding a kettlebell in your right hand in front of your right thigh.
2. Lift your right leg off the floor slightly and find your balance. Once stable, sit your hips backwards and allow your left knee to bend slightly bringing your torso down towards the ground. Your leg can be straight or slightly bent as the right leg goes backwards as your counterbalance. Make sure you keep your back flat and lower yourself until your torso is parallel with the floor.
3. Pause, then drive your weight through the heel of the planted foot back to your starting position. You may need to re-balance between reps. Repeat on the other side.

KB SINGLE ARM SHOULDER PRESS

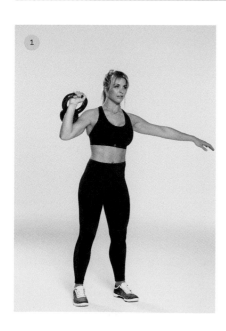

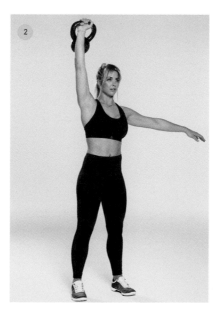

1. Hold the kettlebell by the handle above your shoulder, rotating your wrist as you do so your palm is facing forwards. Set your feet hip-width apart with a slight bend in the knees.
2. Keeping your chest up, shoulder blades back and back straight, drive the kettlebell up towards the ceiling, making sure that when you fully press out the kettlebell is directly above your shoulder joint.
3. Slowly lower the kettlebell back to your starting position and repeat for the set number of reps before changing arms.

3–4

10 REPS PER ARM

40 SECS

WIDE STANCE LEG PRESS

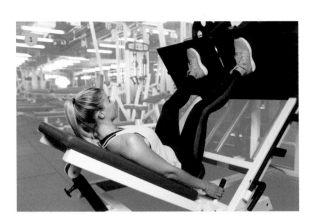

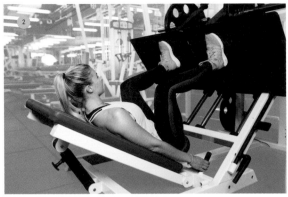

⟳ **3–4**

⏱ **10 REPS**

🏋 **40 SECS**

1. Set yourself into the leg press machine placing your feet just wider than shoulder-width apart, with them slightly turned out towards the top of the foot plate. Press the weight away from you to release the machine or lower yourself into a seated squat position, depending on the type of machine you are using.

2. Lower the weight by flexing the knees and the hips, tracking your knees over your toe line. Do not allow them to collapse inwards. Keep lowering the weight to the bottom of the movement without allowing your lower back to tuck in under you; the pelvis shouldn't move.

3. Pause at the bottom, then drive the weight back up through your heels to the starting position. Do NOT lock the knees at the end range.

CABLE FACE PULLS

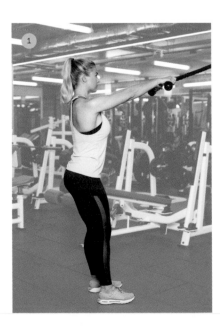

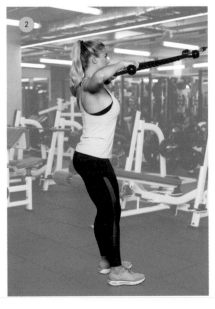

1. Using a high pulley cable machine, attach a rope. Standing feet shoulder-width apart, with back straight and chest up, hold the ends of the rope with an overhand grip.

2. Pull the weight in directly towards your face under control, separating your hands as you do. Keep the upper arms parallel with the floor.

3. Pause just short of your jaw and then return to the starting position. Repeat.

⟳ **3–4**

⏱ **10 REPS**

🏋 **40 SECS**

DB STEP UPS

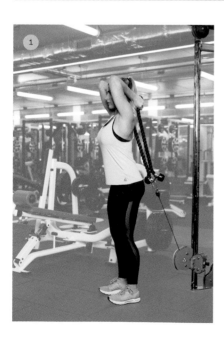

1. Stand upright and hold a set of dumbbells by your sides, palms facing each other. Place your right foot on a solid step that is set at or just above your knee height.
2. Step upwards onto the platform by driving your weight through your heel. Bring yourself fully upright and maintain balance.
3. Step back down slowly with the left leg and repeat for the set number of reps before performing on the other side.

🔄 **3–4**

⏱ **15 REPS PER LEG**

🔋 **40 SECS**

OVERHEAD CABLE TRICEP EXTENSION

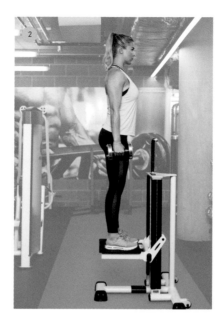

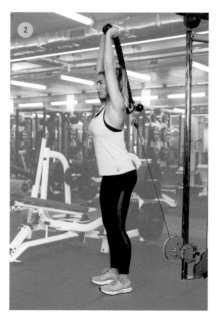

1. Attach a rope to the bottom end of a cable pulley machine. Grab the rope with both hands and extend your arms directly above your head as you face away. Lower your hands towards your shoulder joints. Keep your elbows tight, close to your head, and arms perpendicular to the floor.
2. From this starting position extend your hands up towards the ceiling without the elbows drifting wide and lock the arms out at the tops squeezing the triceps.
3. Pause, then slowly lower the hands back down towards the ground back to your starting position and repeat.

🔄 **3–4**

⏱ **15 REPS**

🔋 **40 SECS**

GYM HIIT, ABS & CORE WORKOUT

WARM UP 5 MINS (PAGE 172)
WORK OUT 35–40 MINS
COOL DOWN 5 MINS (PAGE 176)

Exercise	Sets	Reps or Time	Rest	Target Area
Prowler Sled	5	30 secs	30–45 secs	Cardiovascular Lower Body
Battle Rope Waves	5	30 secs	30–45 secs	Cardiovascular Full Body
Decline Leg Raises	3–4	10–15	30 secs	Abs & Core
Swiss Ball Plank	3–4	20–30 secs	30 secs	Core

 SETS REPS / TIME REST

PROWLER SLED

Load the prowler with roughly 50% of your body weight, i.e. if you weigh 70kg add 35kg to it, or more or less depending how fit / strong you are. Grip the handles at the top of the poles. Bend slightly at the waist, set one foot in front of the other and lock the arms straight. Make sure to keep the spine in its neutral alignment, don't round the back. Working as fast and as hard as you can, push the sled continuously for the set amount of time.

 5

 30 SECS

 30–45 SECS

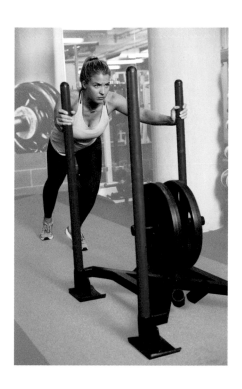

BATTLE ROPE WAVES

From a standing position hold the ends of the ropes at arm's length in front of your hips with your hands shoulder-width apart. Keeping your core tight and back straight with a slight bend in the knees begin alternatively raising and lowering each arm explosively.

 5

 30 SECS

 30–45 SECS

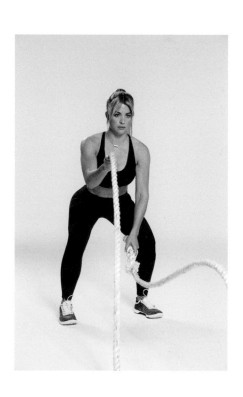

DECLINE LEG RAISES

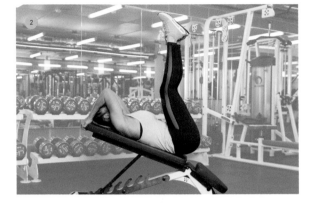

3–4

10–15 REPS

30 SECS

1. Lie with your back on a decline bench with your head towards the highest point. Place your hands above your head holding on to the bench as shown. Your legs should be fully extended but with a slight bend in the knee.
2. Raise your legs in a vertical line position.

3. Under control, lower the legs back down to the starting position and repeat this movement for the set number of reps. This is like the lying leg raises we did in Phase 1 (see page 188), but with increased difficulty. Either adjust the incline or repeat lying on the floor if this is too difficult.

SWISS BALL PLANK

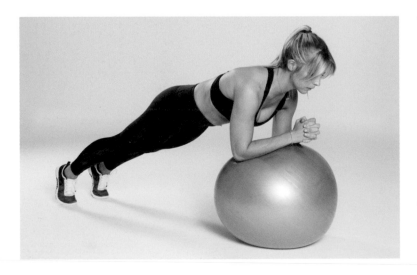

1. Get into a plank position with your elbows on the ball and rest your chest on your forearms with your feet hip-width apart. Once stable, lift your chest up away from the ball so your body weight is now supported by the forearms only. Contract your abs and squeeze your glutes and don't allow your lower back to arch.
2. To challenge your core even further, start to add small hip circles, clockwise and anti-clockwise in a random fashion. If this is too challenging then just hold the plank position for the set amount of time.

 3–4

 20–30 SECS

 30 SECS

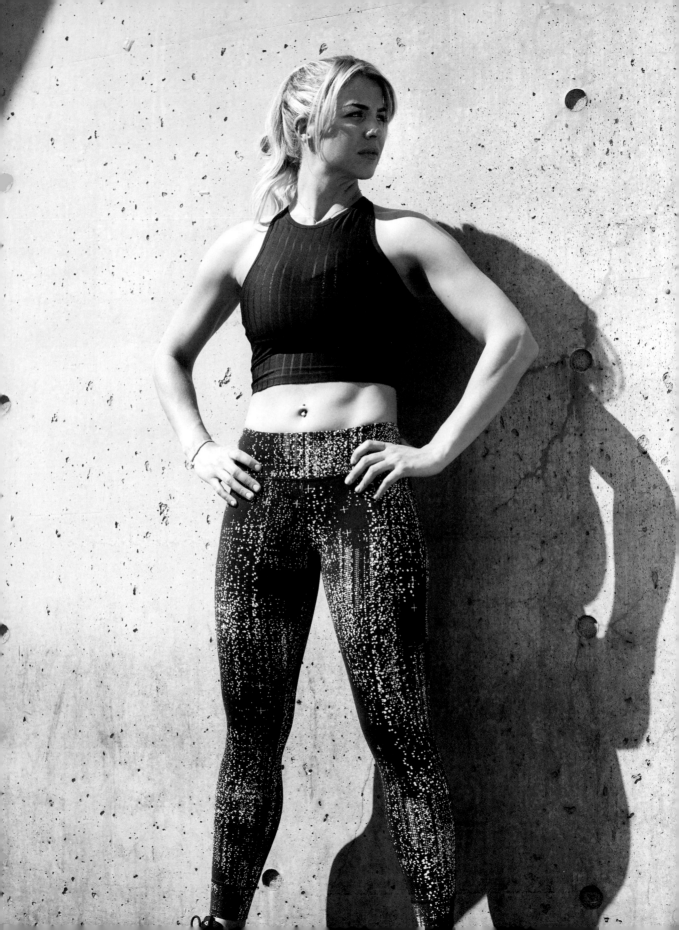

YOUR PROGRESS

Congratulations on completing the Ultimate Body Plan! Whoop! If you've really thrown yourself into this plan – trained hard, eaten right, challenged yourself – you should be feeling leaner, healthier, fitter and so much happier than when you first picked up this book. I am so proud of you and you should be hugely proud of yourself. Making changes is incredibly tough and, even if you have slipped up and cursed my name loudly at stages throughout this process, hopefully you've forgiven both yourself and me now because you have a body you love!

At the start of the plan I asked you to fill out a table detailing your goals, hopes and also worries, and I'm going to ask you to fill out another again now, as a means to measure how far you've come.

Date you finished the plan	
Look back at your objectives from the first table. Did you meet them? Did they change throughout the process?	
How do you feel emotionally having completed the plan?	
How do you feel physically?	
What changes are you most surprised by and proud of?	
Look back at what you said you were most looking forward to experiencing. Can you tick off any of those things already? Have you made plans for ticking them off?	
What were the biggest obstacles you came across?	
How did you overcome these obstacles?	
Look back at the reward your promised yourself – are you going to gift it to yourself now?	
How do you rate how you feel about yourself now, on a scale of 1 – 10, where 1 is 'I don't like myself at all' and 10 is 'I think I'm pretty damn awesome'?	

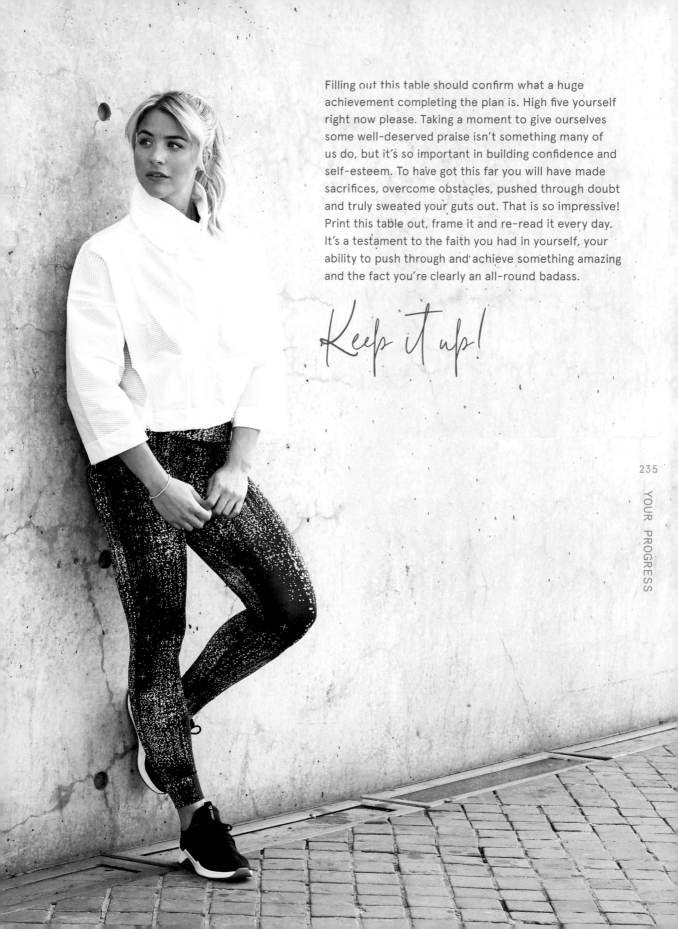

Filling out this table should confirm what a huge achievement completing the plan is. High five yourself right now please. Taking a moment to give ourselves some well-deserved praise isn't something many of us do, but it's so important in building confidence and self-esteem. To have got this far you will have made sacrifices, overcome obstacles, pushed through doubt and truly sweated your guts out. That is so impressive! Print this table out, frame it and re-read it every day. It's a testament to the faith you had in yourself, your ability to push through and achieve something amazing and the fact you're clearly an all-round badass.

Keep it up!

INDEX

RECIPE INDEX

RECICE INDEX CONTINUED

ACKNOWLEDGEMENTS

I'd firstly like to thank the team at HarperCollins, especially Carolyn Thorne who gave me the chance to do this book and finally get my story and message across to people. Thank you to James Empringham, Micaela Alcaino and Sarah Hammond for putting the book together, and to the photography teams for making the shoots so fun and for gorgeous photos: David Cummings, Rowan Spray, Lucy Denver, Martin Poole, Kim Morphew, and Jo Harris.

To Jo Usmar for understanding how I wanted this book to be, and for our long chats about my experiences. It's nice to know I have a voice and a platform that will hopefully inspire others. Thank you to Heather Thomas for help with the delicious recipes.

To Thembi, Bella and Cinta the best glam squad a girl could ask for. Cinta, I genuinely wouldn't have gotten through some situations without you and I will never forget how you made me feel strong again.

To Becca Barr and the whole team at BBM for believing in me for the last 12 years and working with me not only as my agents, but as my friends. I truly feel you are the dream team and I'm so proud to be a small part of it. Here's to many more work ventures!

To Chris and everyone who works with me at Hits Radio. You have given me the freedom and flexibility to do a day job that I love whilst also exploring new ventures and I couldn't be more grateful.

To Jo Hallows who cast me in my role as Lisa Hunter in *Hollyoaks* and the first producer I ever worked for. You got me my foot in the door to this career so thank you for seeing potential in me back then.

To any guy who ever cheated on me or treated me badly. Your bad behaviour helped mould me into the strong woman I am today and taught me what not to accept in relationships. You may have broken my heart temporarily, but you didn't break my spirit or stop me shining.

To my best friends of over 25 years! Laura, Natalie, Marisa, Viki. I have to stay friends with you all, because you bitches know too much ;) From boys, to break-ups, and matching tattoos in Magaluf, from weddings and babies to multiple career changes, we have all stayed true to one another, remained honest and managed to somehow always laugh along the way. I trust you all with all my secrets and I can't wait for us to dance the funky chicken at our 70th birthday parties.

To Evil Steve who isn't really evil at all. He's a genius, a friend and the best PT I have ever worked with. Thanks for everything, and I'm sorry for what I said when I was hungry. Nick Mitchell and the team at UP fitness for always making me feel welcome and part of the team. Keep inspiring fellas! To Olly Foster who first introduced me to weight training. You changed my outlook on my body in a positive way and I'm so thankful.

My incredible family! I love you all so much. Uncle Clive, you have been a constant source of fun in our life from silly jokes to fun trips and chocolates on a Wednesday. Nina, you are the best big sister I could wish for. Losing Dad without you there meant I would have lost myself, you helped bring me back to life and pushed me to move forward through the most painful experience. I also love that we have the same size feet because you have nicer shoes than me. Rob, my brother-in-law, thank you for taking care of my sister and my nephews and niece. They are so lucky to have a dad like you. Mum and Peter, I couldn't function without you. It's only as an adult I realise what a strong woman you are, Mum, and you inspire me to be the same. I hope to one day be half the mum that you are. You taught me to never quit, never lose sight of what's important and to never just settle. Peter, from doing DIY jobs around my house to always listening when I needed advice, and for making my mum so happy.

To Norman and Ollie my amazing doggies! Having you both taught me to have responsibility for something other than myself and you always make me smile, even after you both had the shits all over my kitchen floor that time. I've always said humans don't deserve dogs and it's true.

To Gorka, my love and my best friend. Thank you for showing me that happy endings do indeed exist. For loving me, supporting me, comforting me when I need it most, reminding me of what truly matters in life and for always being up for any kind of adventure with me. You make me feel like the most beautiful woman every single day and although every love story is amazing, ours is my favourite.

Lastly, my dad, David. You won't get to read this, but I know that throughout all of the stories in this book, you have been present watching over me and keeping me safe. Living more than half of my life without you in it has been hard at times, but the 17 years we did have, I hold fondly in my heart and I will never forget how you loved me, what hopes you had for me, how hard you worked to provide for me and our conversation the last time you saw me. I hope I've made you proud, Dad.

If you have experienced a bereavement as a child or young adult and need support, please contact Grief Encounter on 020 8371 8455 or support@griefencounter.org.uk. For more information on the charity, visit griefencounter.org.uk